AF564859

A Fully Illustrated Handbook on Clinical Diagnostic Processes in Canine Medicine

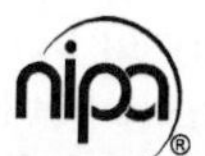

NIPA® GENX ELECTRONIC RESOURCES & SOLUTIONS P. LTD.
New Delhi-110 034

About the Authors

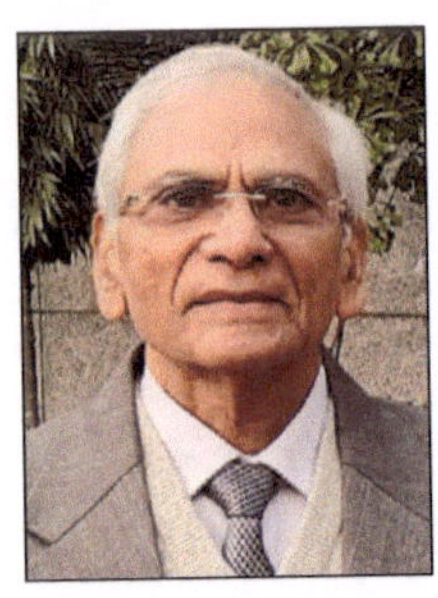

Prof. (Dr.) J.P. Varshney, Former Principal Scientist (Veterinary Medicine, ICAR-IVRI, Izatnagar), with a vast clinical, research and teaching experience of more than 57 years, is still continuing his dedicated yeoman clinical services at Nandini Veterinary Hospital, Surat (Gujarat). His work in animal electrocardiography and cardiology is well recognized and earned him reputation. He has been bestowed with Dr. K.S. Nair Memorial Gold Medal—1990, Dr. C.G. Bhaskar Gold Medal—1996, Ram Lal Agrawal Gold Medal—1997, Award of Merit-2001 (ICAR-IVRI,Izatnagar), Award of Honour-2002 (ICAR-IVRI,Izatnagar), Best Teacher Award 2003-2004 (ICAR-IVRI, Izatnagar), PETCARE Award for Canine Excellence-2005, Dr. C.M. Singh Memorial Lifetime Achievement Award-2020, VIPM Lifetime Achievement Award -2021 and an honour of "Living Legend of Homeopathy-2023" (3rd Homeopathy Vijnana Sammelan, Ahmedabad) besides many other honors and awards. Apart from publications in national/international scientific journals of repute, he is the author of books namely "Equine Parasitic Diseases and Their Management (ICAR-IVRI Izatnagar Publication, 2003), "Research Findings -Homeopathic Bio efficacy and Management of Animal Health (Sintex International Limited, Kalol, Gujarat 2007) , "Electrocardiography in Veterinary Medicine" (Springer Nature, Singapore, 2020), "Handbook of Exotic Pet Medicine" (Brillion Publishing, New Delhi, 2021), "Ultrasound in Veterinary Medicine: Fundamentals and Applications " (NIPA, New Delhi,2022), and "Heart Failure in Animals: Current Concepts" (NIPA, New Delhi,2023)

A Fully Illustrated Handbook on Clinical Diagnostic Processes in Canine Medicine

J.P. Varshney B.V.Sc. and A.H.; M.V.Sc. (Veterinary Medicine)
Ph.D. (Veterinary Medicine.)
Ex. Principal Scientist (Veterinary Medicine, IVRI Izatnagar)
Senior Consultant (Veterinary Medicine)
Nandini Veterinary Hospital
Ghod-Dod Road, Surat-395001, Gujarat, India

NIPA® GENX ELECTRONIC RESOURCES & SOLUTIONS P. LTD.
New Delhi-110 034

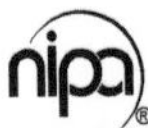

NIPA® GENX ELECTRONIC RESOURCES & SOLUTIONS P. LTD.

101,103, Vikas Surya Plaza, CU Block
L.S.C. Market, Pitam Pura, New Delhi-110 034
Ph : +91 11 27341616, 27341717, 27341718
E-mail: newindiapublishingagency@gmail.com
Website: www.nipabooks.com
For customer assistance, please contact
Phone: + 91-11-27 34 17 17
Fax: + 91-11-27 34 16 16
E-Mail: feedbacks@nipabooks.com

Print ISBN: 978-93-58879-97-1

ebook ISBN: 978-93-58874-47-1

Composed and Designed by NIPA®.

Dedicated to
My Late Parents
(Smt. Ramwati Devi and Devi Ram Varshney)
and
Teachers

Acknowledgements

I profusely thank my better half, Jai Prabha Varshney, who has always stood with me with all her positivity in odd and even times. Emotional support, care and concern of my daughters (Pratibha, Ritu and Prabhanshi), sons (Atul, Prabhat and Ajit), and grandchildren (Agrima, Vedaant, Devansh and Anvi) had been encouraging in accomplishing this task.

Help rendered by Dr. Hardik Monapara, my colleague, is duly acknowledged. I would like to thank Shri Nayan N. Bharatia - Managing Trustee and Board of Trustees, Nandini Veterinary Hospital, Surat for their encouragement and support for greater cause of extending knowledge among professionals engaged in animal health care.

I shall fail in my duty if I do not acknowledge contribution of my patients who were instrumental in providing material and ideas to be translated in the form of this book.

(J.P.Varshney)

Preface

As a custodian of animal health, Veterinarians are charged with the responsibility of making an early and correct diagnosis so that health care interventions can be undertaken well in time. Since inception of health care, diagnosis (understanding the disease and its pathogenesis) has been in the core of all health care systems throughout the world whether it is human health care (Ayurveda, Allopathy, Homeopathy, Chinese medicine, Unani medicine , etc.) or animal health care (Veterinary Medicine) as it provides an explanation of health problems and assists in taking subsequent health care decisions. In earlier days, information gathering through conversation and physical examination of the patient had been the basis of making diagnosis. With the passage of time, development and inclusion of new techniques of examination have revolutionized the process of making diagnosis. The specialty of canine medicine is following the foot prints of human medicine in adopting the diagnostic techniques as well as newer therapeutic developments because of owners' willingness for an excellent health care of their beloved pets on the pattern of human medicine. In routine practice, clinical manifestations such as anorexia, diarrhea, fever, weakness, ascites, liver disease, lameness, vomiting, anemia, swelling, epistaxis, hematuria, salivation, ataxia etc. are inadvertently mistaken as diagnoses. Diagnostic misconceptions such as hypothyroidism or euthyroidism, stroke or syncope, fever or hyperthermia, seizure/syncope, paresis or paralysis, vomiting or regurgitation, cough or vomitus are also rampant in canine practice. Such casual or symptomatic diagnoses have negative health outcome. Unnecessary use of polypharmacy or irrational drugs increases metabolic load on body, delays recovery, increases illness period, delays potentially lifesaving treatment, and causes psychological distress and financial burden on owners .While accurate and timely diagnosis has positive impact on health outcome as clinical decision are tailored according to correct understanding of the health problem. In fact diagnosis of any ailment is identification of the underlying disease and disease process correlating it with clinical manifestations with an understanding of its etiology and its impact on structure and functions of the body. A comprehensive process of diagnosis involves history taking to provide leads, general physical examination to determine functional abnormality, special examination of a suspected compromised organ or system(s), special examination of an affected system to locate lesion, special examination of the lesion to specify its nature and special examination of specimen (biopsy) to determine the cause. The important pillars of the diagnosis are history and clinical examination; knowledge and application of diagnostic techniques; and laboratory examination including the use of diagnostics, hematological panel, metabolic profile, organ function tests, acid- base and gas analysis, immunological tests, microbial culture and sensitivity test etc.. The first two aspects of the disease diagnosis process are in the domain of clinician who can effectively contribute to the process of diagnosis. In the absence of subjective symptoms in animals, a systematic physical examination assumes greater responsibility. Before proceeding to make any examination of the patient, it is necessary to take into account the owner's complaint, patient's detail , environmental history, diet and habits, vaccination status, deworming status, disease history along with treatment details if any. The description of the patient with regard to species, breed, age, sex is a useful part in identifying the patient and in assisting diagnosis. Palpation, percussion and auscultation are integral part of clinical examination. The results of physical or clinical examinations heavily depend on the knowledge of the clinician with respect to anatomy, physiology, pathology, animal behavior, skills in the methods and technique of examination, clinical signs and disease pathogenesis. The other complementary steps, however, requires specific techniques and laboratory investigations.

Nowadays, traditional bedside evaluation skills (history and physical examination) are being underutilized due to over reliance and large growth of diagnostic techniques which are being considered one of the fundamental pillars of modern medicine. Sometimes over-reliance on instrumental techniques leads to over diagnosis. These techniques with all their advantages cannot replace or undermine the importance of physical examination conducted by an experienced clinician as these techniques provide 2nd round of information to refine the diagnostic process. It is therefore necessary that all the pillars of diagnostic process are given due weightage and a comprehensive systematic approach is adopted while examining the patient.

The book "A Fully Illustrated Handbook on Clinical Diagnostic Processes in Canine Medicine" aims at improving the clinical diagnostic skill of veterinarians (novice veterinary students, veterinary graduates, veterinary practitioners and scholars) engaged in canine practice with respect to first two basic components of diagnostic process (history and physical examination) and making familiar with diagnostic protocol in relation to diseases of various body systems. The book does not claim to provide comprehensive knowledge regarding radiography, electrocardiography, echocardiography, ultrasonography, endoscopy, MRI, CT scan, encephalography, ophthalmoscopy etc. to make readers expert as these techniques are specialties in itself and are beyond the scope of this book. Nevertheless, basic preliminary knowledge about these techniques has been given to acquaint the readers with the indications, merits and limitations of these advance techniques so that cases, requiring intervention of these techniques, are timely referred to appropriate subject matter specialist.

It is anticipated that the book will serve its purpose of making readers familiar with clinical diagnostic process and improving their clinical acumen so that bedside diagnosis does not remain underutilized.

(J.P.Varshney)

Contents

1

Diagnosis and Diagnostic Process

Veterinarian's primary responsibility towards patients and their owners is to establish a correct diagnosis as it is a pre-requisite for rational, effective, eco-friendly and cheap treatment. Diagnosis of a disease is the crux of health problems. An accurate and prompt diagnosis helps in deciding effective treatment options, whereas incorrect and delayed diagnosis often leads to failure in disease outcome.

Diagnosis

The word "diagnosis" is derived from the Greek word "gnosis" that means knowledge. The diagnosis is not only the identification of the disease but also of disease process correlating with clinical manifestations with an understanding of disease etiology and its influence on the structure and function of the body. In fact making diagnosis is itself a process of ascertaining the nature of the disease or disorder from its signs and symptoms differentiating it from similar looking conditions. Ascertaining the cause of illness in dogs and cats is not an easy task as many diseases have similar clinical symptoms. In health care, diagnosis is most important process since the protocol for therapeutic intervention solely depends on this step. Diagnosis of the ailments depends on clinical reasoning and should be accurate and timely. Reliability of diagnosis is essential in health care. It becomes all the more important in case of infectious diseases as undiagnosed or under diagnosed pets may spread the infection to others.

In routine practice diagnoses are generally made as anorexia, fever, loose motion, ascites, weakness, vomiting, panting, shivering, ataxia, anemia, nasal bleeding etc. In fact these are not diagnoses but are the clinical manifestations of underlying disease/s and therefore require the identification of the underlying disease and disease process. Such casual diagnoses may prevent or delay appropriate treatment, may lead to administration of unnecessary medicines, may cause delayed recovery, and may cause psychological trauma to owner with financial repercussion.

Making a correct and an early diagnosis is very much important for undertaking rational and effective treatment for fast recovery, avoiding unnecessary medication, reducing the load of so many drugs on body metabolism, reducing environmental pollution and the cost of treatment. There are four important pillars (Fig .1) for making a correct diagnosis viz. the history, the systematic clinical examination, the correct clinical diagnostic techniques and the laboratory support. Broadly speaking the diagnosis is an amalgamation of history, clinical manifestations, clinical examination of the patient, examination of environment, special examinations using electrocardiography, echocardiography, Doppler echocardiography, electroencephalography, ultrasonography, endoscopy, radiography, tomography, image intensification, scintigraphy and laboratory tests as per the merit of the case . There has been a considerable emphasis on the clinical, instrumental and laboratory diagnosis of the individual animal affected with the disease. Prof. Well and Halsled (1967) rightly stated "A Clinician who depends much on laboratory to make his diagnosis is probably inexperienced; one who says that he does not need instruments or a laboratory is uninformed" Therefore, clinical examination including history, application of diagnostic tools and laboratory are complementary to each other.

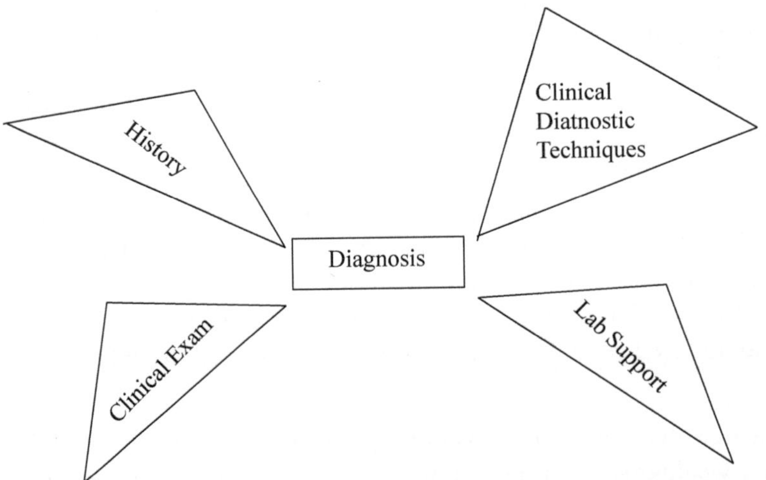

Figure 1: Pillars of Diagnosis. Making a correct diagnosis depends on examination of history, physical examination of the patient, correct use of relevant diagnostic techniques as well as laboratory examination in relation of clinical observations.

Important Developments in Clinical Diagnostic Techniques

- In the past, clinicians and veterinarians depended heavily on the history, observations and examinations for making diagnosis.

- Invention of compound microscope in the end of 16th century made a great headway in the diagnosis of diseases.
- Another advancement in diagnostic techniques was the invention of thermometer in 1714 by German physicist Daniel Fahrenheit.
- Invention of stethoscope by French Physician Rene-theophile-Hyacinthe Laennec in 1816 improved the ability of physicians and veterinarians to diagnose diseases of heart and chest.
- In 1850 development of ophthalmoscope by Hermann von Helmholtz, a German scientist, facilitated the diagnosis of eye diseases.
- First human electrocardiogram was recorded by Augustus Waller in May, 1887. Since then it has facilitated the diagnosis of cardiac arrhythmias.
- Year 1895 witnessed the discovery of greatest anatomic diagnostic tool "X-ray" by German physicist Wilhelm Conrad Rontgen. It has revolutionized the imaging of internal organs of the body.
- In 1942 Karl Dussik used ultrasonography for the first time in medical diagnoses. Since then it has become an important diagnostic technique for imaging internal organs.
- First echocardiogram was taken by Inge Edler and C. Hellmuth Hertz in 1953. It has now facilitated the differential diagnosis of cardiomyopathies, vulvular diseases, pericardial effusions etc.
- During early 1970, introduction of computed tomography (CT) has increased the scope and safety of imaging procedures allowing to view the arrangement and functioning of body's internal structures.
- Introduction of PET (Positron Emission Tomography) scan facilitated measuring cell activity in organs.
- During 1990 CAT (computed axial tomography) or CT (computed tomography) has found its use in the diagnosis and characterization of certain cancers, heart diseases and studying the brain.

Diagnostic process

Diagnosis is the end point of complex process centered on the patient, collaborating with patient as well as other sources of gathering information such as clinical history, physical examination, examination employing diagnostic techniques and laboratory information.

Physical Examination

Physical /clinical examination is a fundamental part of the process of diagnosis .It is routinely done to diagnose diseases in dogs and cats presented in the clinics .Physical examination provides important information needed for determining the disease or diseases producing the clinical abnormalities. Information gathered during physical/clinical examination of the ailing dogs /cats assist in determining the organs/system involved, type and location of the lesion, pathophysiological process and severity of the disease. Results of physical examination depends heavily on the knowledge of the clinician regarding anatomy, physiology, pathology and animal behavior as well as his skills in the methods and techniques of clinical examination, recognizing clinical sign and understanding of disease pathogenesis. Without a proficient physical examination, an accurate diagnosis is unlikely leading to treatment failure.

Clinician first step in making a diagnosis is through asking the owners' complaint. Accurate and complete history may be obtained from focusing on the details of the patient (species, breed, age , sex, name, weight), vaccination status, deworming schedule, nutritonal history, past and present medical history and environmental history. Physical examination of the patient involves general inspection, palpation, percussion, and auscultation to detect manifestations of abnormalities.

Physical Examination Techniques

- General observations- It starts as soon as clinician sees his/her patient. Patients' general condition, gait, posture, mentation and behavior is noted without disturbing the patient.
- Palpation- Palpation (Figure 2) is the technique that aims at ascertaining the size, shape, consistency, and temperature of the area/organ under examination. Palpation can be done using the fingers (direct palpation) or using a probe (indirect palpation). Palpation may be light or deep. In light palpation tissue/organ is felt gently. While in deep palpation, more pressure is applied to obtain information about the consistency of the tissue or to detect pain or to feel abdominal organs.

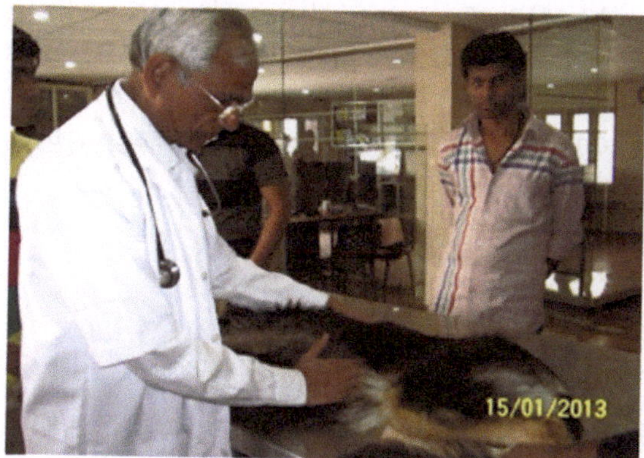

Figure 2: Showing the technique of palpation using finger tips.

- Percussion- It is the method of examination (Figure3) in which body parts are tapped with fingers, hands or small instruments to determine the size, consistency and borders of the organs; and to ascertain the presence or absence of the fluid in the body. The tapping of the area/organ elicits a sound. Percussion sounds help us in differentiating whether the organ is air filled (as lungs), dense (as liver) or fluid filled (as urinary bladder). The air filled organs such as lungs produce hollow low pitched resonance. Solid organs, bones and joints produce dull sound as is produced on percussion of liver. Percussion of fluid (urinary bladder) or fluid with air filled organs (stomach, intestines) produce tympanic high pitched drum like longer duration resonance.

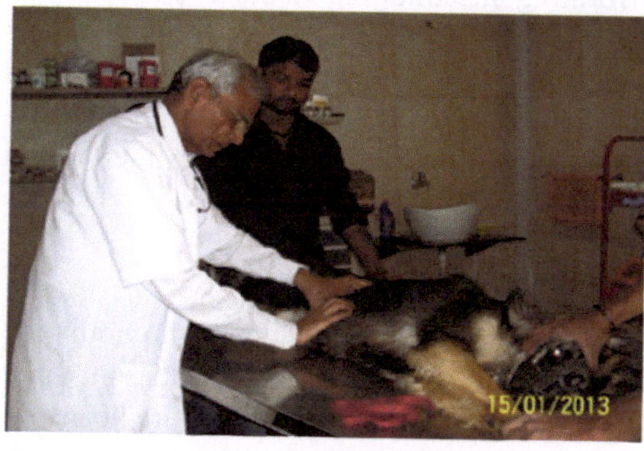

Figure 3: Showing the technique of percussion

- Auscultation- The word "auscultate" is derived from a Latin word "Auscultare" that means "Listen". Auscultation is still an important diagnostic technique of listening sounds of internal body organs such as heart, lungs and intestines either directly (putting the ear directly on heart area or chest) or indirectly using an instrument called "Stethoscope". Stethoscope was invented in France in 1816 by Rene Theophile Hyacinthe Laennec. It is composed of chest piece, diaphragm, bell, tubing, stem, head set, ear tubes and ear pieces (Figure4).

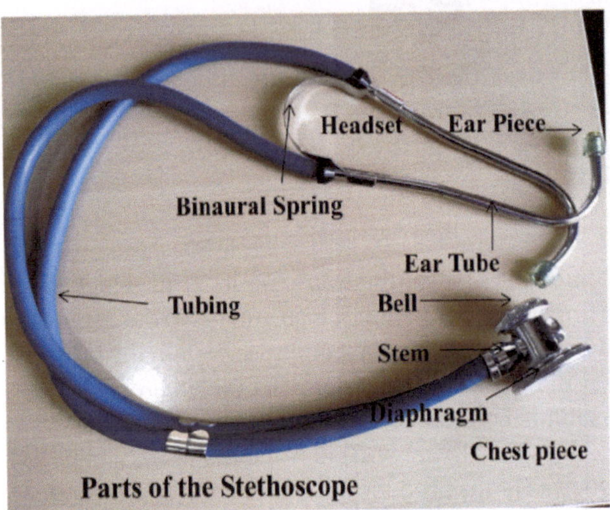

Figure 4: Showing different parts of the stethoscope.

The pet should be relaxed in a quiet room before auscultation is performed to avoid disturbing humming sounds. It is advisable to perform auscultation in a standing position. .While performing auscultation, stethoscope should be pressed firmly (not too hard) on the area to be auscultated to avoid sound of hair scratching on the diaphragm of the stethoscope. For better results auscultation should be performed by placing stethoscope at least five locations (4th, 6th, 8th intercostals space at two third height of the thorax ; 4th and 6th intercostals space at one third height of the thorax) on each side of the thorax.

(i) Lung Auscultation

It provides valuable information. The lungs are auscultated on the both side of the thorax in the area shown in the Figure 5 .On thorax auscultation, three types of sounds (extra thoracic, pleural and broncho-pulmonary) are heard.

Extra thoracic sounds are caused by the movement of the stethoscope tubing on the hairs or trembling of the muscle. Pleural rubbings are heard in cases of pleuritis owing to pleural movements. Pleural rubbing sounds are generally not heard in dogs and cats because pleuritis is exudative in these animals rather than fibrinous.

Normal bronchopulmonary sounds may be inaudible, weaker, of normal loudness only during inspiration, or louder. The character of respiratory sound is almost similar to those heard over the trachea (inspiration and expiration are alike). In general, respiratory pattern and lung sounds are subtle in cats as compared to dogs. The normal breath sounds can be divided into three categories such as bronchial breath sounds, bronchiovascular breath sound and vesicular breath sound. Bronchial breath sounds are strong and relatively harsh blowing sound heard over the trachea and hilar region. Inspiratory and expiratory components of bronchial sounds are prominent. Bronchiovascular sounds have both inspiratory (soft) and expiratory (short but more prominent than vesicular sound) character and are intermediate between bronchial and vesicular sounds. Vesicular sound is normal lung sound and is heard in the periphery of lung. Vesicular sound consists of soft inspiratory and a soft short expiratory sounds.

Adventitious sounds are abnormal lung sounds and indicate lung pathology. These sounds are of two types viz. discontinuous and continuous. Crackles (rales) are discontinuous explosive sounds associated with lung edema. Crackles heard throughout inspiration indicate disease of large airways. Whereas crackles heard at the end of inspiration are suggestive of small airways disease. Crackles can be low pitch (associated with airways secretions), high pitch (associated with opening of collapsed peripheral airways) or pleural friction rub (low pitched associated with roughened pleural surfaces). Wheezes are continuous sounds with musical character associated with asthma or bronchitis. Wheezes heard during expiration are due to dynamic compression of airways. When wheezes are heard at the end of inspiration are suggestive of opening of smaller inflamed airways. Stridor is another abnormal continuous monophonic musical sound primarily heard during inspiration. It is associated with laryngeal or tracheal disease. Stertor is snoring sound without musical character. It is harsh continuous crackling sound in trachea or larynx due to edema and accumulation of secretions in upper airways.

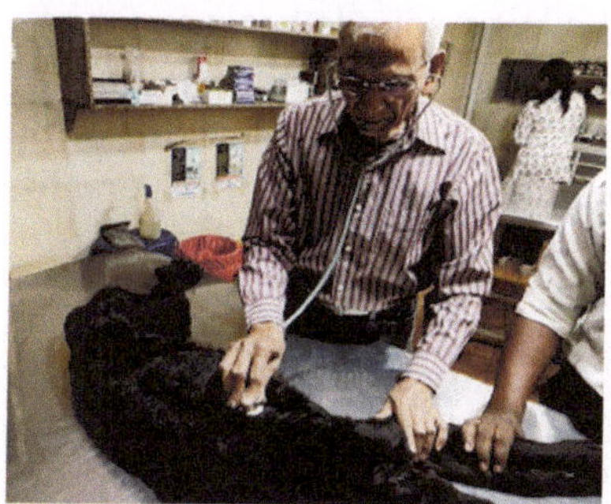
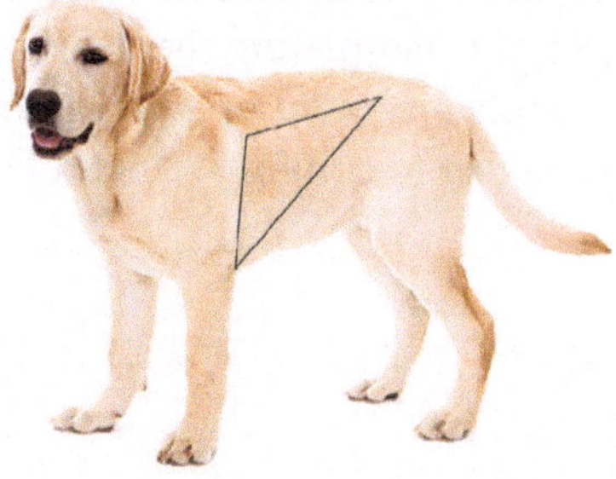

Figure 5. Area marked for auscultation of lungs on both side of the thorax.

(ii) Cardiac Auscultation

Cardiac auscultation is an important part of clinical examination as it gives information about rate and rhythm of the heart; presence or absence of cardiac murmurs and muffling of heart sound. Heart sound is characterized by LUB-DUB-PAUSE. Sound of LUB (S1) is associated with closure of mitral and tricuspid valves. While sound of DUB (S2) is associated with closure of aortic and pulmonary valves.

Auscultation of the heart should be done in a quiet room with relaxed dog/cat in standing position at apex, at base and at the level of all valves' (mitral, tricuspid, aortic and pulmonary). The pet should be gently restrained and the clinician should also be relaxed. These conditions for auscultation matters much. A cat can be restrained gently with one hand under the abdomen. Ventilation artifacts can be reduced by gently holding the mouth close. Showing the cat water in sink or gently pressing over the larynx has been reported to reduce the degree of purring in cat. Mitral, aortic and pulmonary valves are auscultated on the left side of the thorax in standing position at 5th intercostal space around costo-chondral junction (opposite to elbow point in standing position), at 4th intercostal space dorsal to mitral valve (at the level of the point of shoulder), and at 3rd intercostal space at sternal border respectively (Fig .6). Tricuspid valve (Figure6) is auscultated on the right side of the thorax at 3rd to 4th intercostal space at costo-chondral junction. In cats, mitral valve and pulmonic valves are auscultated on the left side at 5th/6th intercostal space above the sternum, and at 2nd/3rd intercostal space one third of the way up from sternum respectively. The tricuspid valve in the cat is auscultated on the right side of the thorax at 4th/5th intercostal space near sternum. Heart sounds are more intense in young dogs, thin/emaciated dogs as well as in disease conditions such as fever, anemia, or hyperthyroidism. Obesity, pleural effusion or pericardial effusion decreases the intensity of the normal heart sounds. Muffled heart sounds (decrease intensity of heart sounds) may be due to pericardial effusion, pericarditis, pleural effusion, diaphragmatic hernia, thoracic neoplasia, hypothyroidism or cardiac temponade. Obesity can also muffle the heart sounds because fat acts as an insulting layer dampening the heart sounds. In dogs, pericardial effusion results from neoplastic or idiopathic diseases. While pericardial effusion in cats is most often due to congestive heart failure secondary to cardiomyopathy.

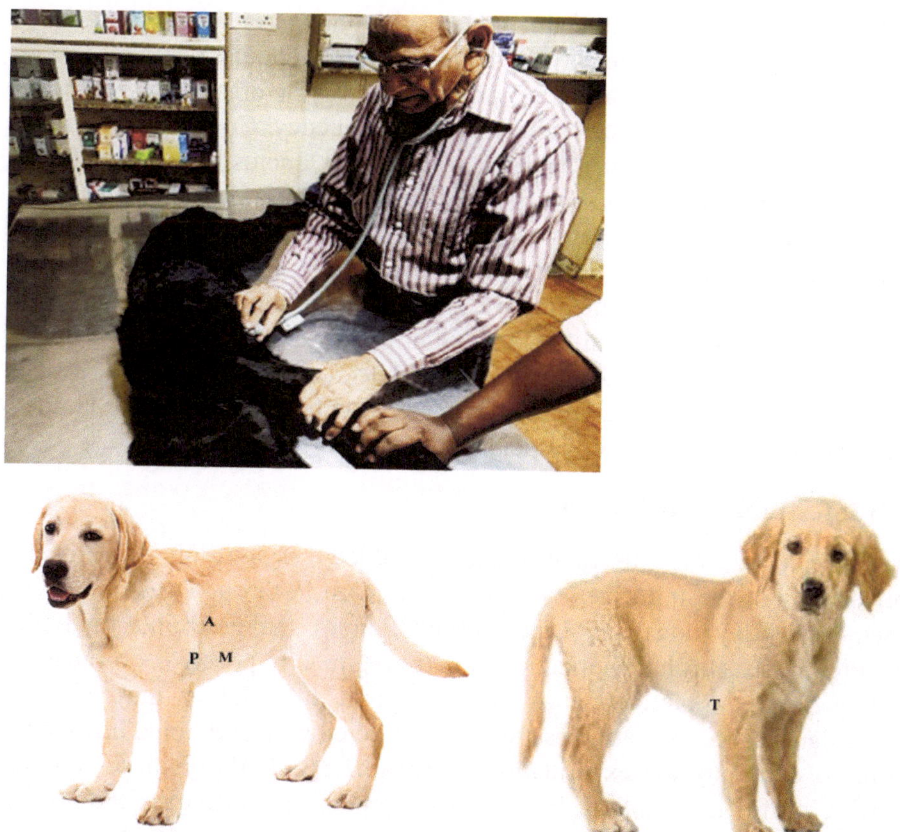

Figure 6: Location of the heart valves in dogs for auscultation. On left side of the thorax P, A and M indicates pulmonary valve , aortic valve and mitral valve respectively. Pulmonary valve (P) is auscultated at 3rd intercostal space near the elbow just above sternum. Aortic valve (A) is auscultated slightly dorsal and caudal to Pulmonary valve at 4th intercostal space. Mitral valve (M) is auscultated slightly caudal and ventral to Aortic valve at 5th intercostal space. On the right side of the thorax T indicates tricuspid valve. It is auscultated at 3th /4th intercostal space near costochondral junction.

Heart murmurs are abnormal, extra, unusual sounds of relatively long duration in the heart beat, generated owing to turbulence within heart due to disturbance in blood flow. Murmurs are also audible in physiological conditions such as in young growing animals even in the absence of any heart disease (generally resolved with growth of the animal); anemia and hypoproteinemia; as well as in cardiac diseases such as valvular insufficiency, valvular stenosis, interatrial or intraventricular septal defects, patent ductus arteiosus or defect of great vessels. Murmurs are categorized as systolic (occurring during systole), diastolic (occurring during diastole) or continuous (occurring during systole and diastole i.e. occurring all time) as per the timings of their occurrence at the point of maximum intensity. Systolic murmurs are quite common and are of soft nature occurring during an early systole. While diastolic murmurs are of less common occurrence and are of low frequency. Continuous murmurs vary in intensity and are associated with patent ductus arteriosus (PDA). Depending on intensity, murmurs have been graded into 6 grades (grade 1 to grade 6). Grade 1 murmurs are soft and localized barely audible. Grade 2 murmurs are similar to grade 1 murmurs but are easily audible. Grade 3 murmurs are moderately intense and are detected at more than one location. Grade 4 murmurs are similar to grade 3 murmurs except that they are detected at many places in left and right thorax. Grade 5 murmurs are loud at point of maximum intensity and are also associated with precordial thrill. Grade 6 murmurs are loudest and are associated with precordial thrill.

(iii) Intestinal Auscultation

Borborygmi are the intestinal sounds, produced as a result of peristaltic movements of the intestines that propel the digesta through gastrointestinal tract, in healthy dogs and cats. Auscultation of the gastrointestinal tract (Figure7) assists in characterization of borborygmi as hypoactive, normoactive or hyperactive. Characterization of borborygmi, in isolation, may not have much significance. Nevertheless, when considered with additional history and results of other physical examinations, the character of borborygmi sounds may provide useful information. Hyperactive borborygmi in diarrheic dogs/cats with losing weight may be suggestive of malabsorption syndrome. Hypoactive borborygmi in dogs/cats with vomiting may be suggestive of gastrointestinal obstruction. Complete absence of borborygmi is indicative of paralytic ileus.

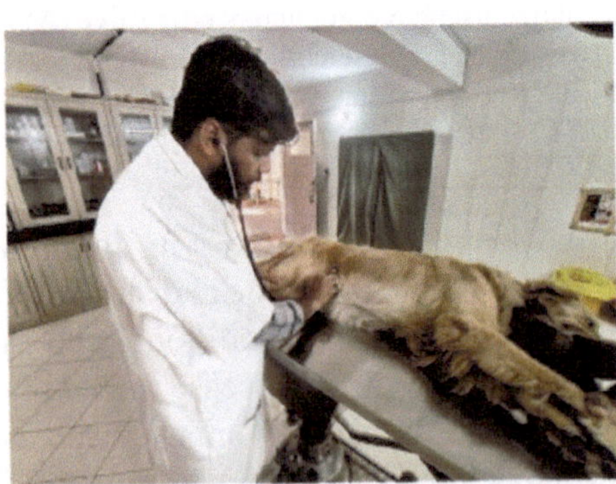

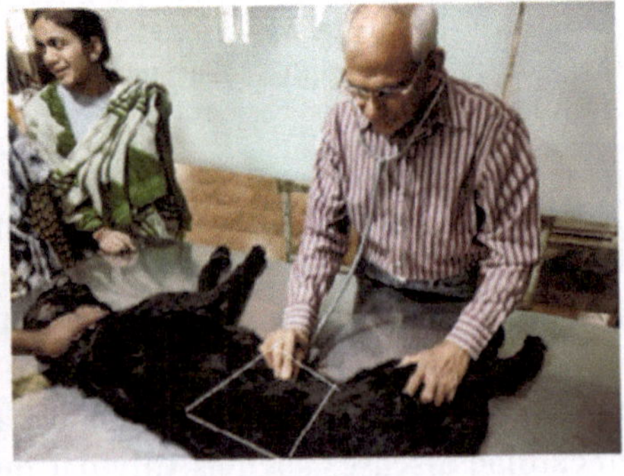

Figure 7: Auscultation of intestines on the right abdomen in a dog. Area for auscultation is marked by white lines.

Steps in Physical Examination

1. *Signalment*: It is about complete details of the patient such as name of the patient, species, breed, age, sex, body weight, reproductive status, distinguishing characteristics, owner's name and address with mobile number. Data of the pet patient is essential to identify the patient.

2. *History Taking*: History taking is a process of getting valuable detailed information about the illness of the patient through careful questioning the owner. In canine/feline practice, disease is presented indirectly in the form of complaint by the owner or attendant of the pet. Many times, owner or attendant fails to provide relevant and adequate information leading to misdiagnosis. It is imperative on the part of the clinician to ask rational questions utilizing his professional knowledge and experience.

History includes information about environment, diet, past medical history including drugs being given, allergies, reproductive history, vaccination status, deworming status, life style of the pet, and main presenting complaint , its genesis and duration. Questioning of the owner should be in such a way that useful information is derived. Instead of asking directly as "Whether the dog had diarrhea?", it will be more meaningful to ask as "Have you seen stool of the pet" What was its color, consistency and frequency? This will help the clinician to ascertain whether the patient had diarrhea or not.

3. *General Appearance:* The dog/cat is observed from a distance as well as closely for symmetry, size and shape of extremities, gait/posture, general looks, body condition (obese or emaciated), hydration and mentation (level of consciousness, alertness, responsiveness), before it is handled. Hydration status is classed as adequate, marginal or inadequate. Skin loses its elasticity (skin turgor) in dehydration. It is measured as the time skin tenting (Figure8) persists. Skin tenting test is conducted on the skin of upper eye lid (Figure8 A) or neck (Figure8 B) by gently pulling up the skin and then letting the skin go. If the skin quickly bounces back and becomes flat, it indicates normal hydration status. Skin may tent more in emaciated animals .It is difficult to perform skin tenting test on obese animals as they may not show tenting even when dehydrated.

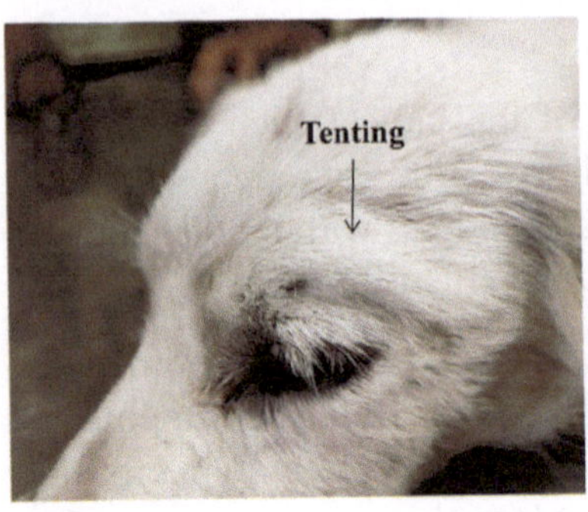

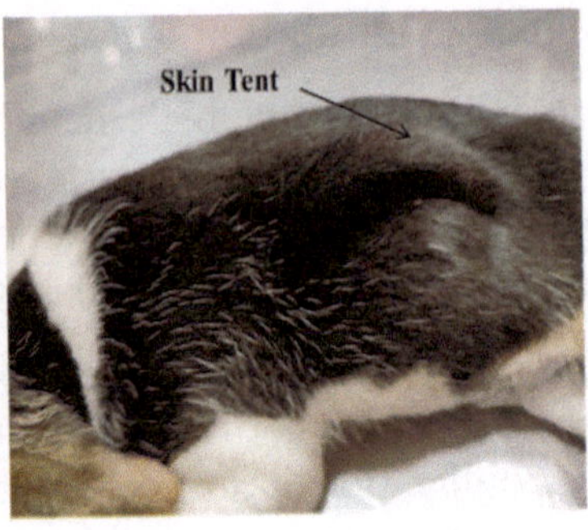

A B

Figure 8: (A) Showing skin tenting in dogs on the skin of upper eye lid **(B)** and on the skin.

4. *Evaluation of Vital signs:* Evaluate body weight, rectal temperature, pulse rate and its character, respiratory rate and its character, mucus membrane color, skin tenting and capillary refill time.

Rectal temperature is recorded by inserting the lubricated digital thermometer into the rectum at an angle that it touches mucus membrane and keeping it for specified time (Figure 9). Digital thermometers are timed and sound when an accurate temperature is obtained. Take out the thermometer, wipe off lubricant and feces and read the temperature. Clean the thermometer with disinfectant (alcohol). Generally avoid mercury thermometers because their breaking may expose the dog/cat to injury and toxic mercury. Rectal temperature of healthy dogs (100.5 to 102.5^{0}F) and cats (98.1 to 102.1^{0}F) is variable. Dogs and cats with rectal temperature beyond specified limit needs to be evaluated further.

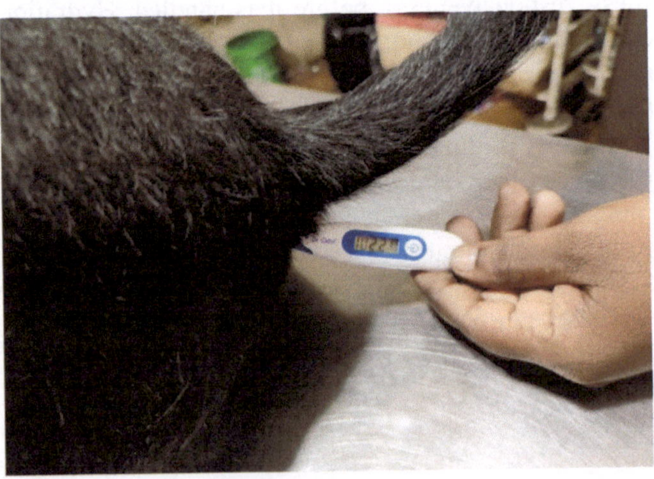

Figure 9: Showing the process of taking temperature in a dog. The thermometer in inserted into the rectum and is tilted slightly upward so that it is in contact with mucus membrane.

Pulse rate is generally taken at femoral artery. Pulse is evaluated for rate, strength and quality (weak, thread, strong, bounding). Compare pulse of both sides' femoral artery and heart rate. If pulse rate is less than heart rate, it indicates pulse deficit and further investigations are warranted. Pulse rate varies from 60 to 160 per minute in healthy dogs (60-120/minute in large dogs and 120 to 160/ minute in small dogs) ; and from 160 to 200 /minute in healthy adult cats. Irregular pulse is indicative of arrhythmias. Bounding pulse (increased pulse pressure) is seen in hyper dynamic (compensatory) state of shock. Weak pulse in seen in patients with decreased cardiac output, peripheral vasoconstriction, thrombosis or decreased pulse pressure. Decreased pulse rate or bradycardia (decreased heart rate) is due to decreased cardiac output and subsequent poor perfusion. Cats with shock may develop bradycardia. Tachycardia (> 180 bpm dogs, > 220 bpm cats) is associated with compromised diastolic filling, hypovolemic shock, pain, hyperthermia or primary cardiac disease.

Resting respiration rate is taken by watching a resting dog or cat taking a breath in (inhaling) and then out (exhaling). Count the breaths in one minute. If number of breaths are counted for 30 seconds then multiply the breath number by 2 for getting the respiratory rate in one minute. Respiration rate can also be determined by lung auscultation. In general normal dogs and cats have respiration rate of 15 to 30 per minutes.

Perfusion indicators includes color of the mucus membranes and capillary refill time. Color of the mucus membrane is determined by visual observation of the mucus membrane. Color of the mucus membrane is the indicative of blood flow to peripheral tissues. In healthy pets, mucus membranes are pink and moist. Cats mucus membranes are little paler than dogs. Sometimes mucus membrane color changes are subtle and may not correlate with significant medical condition. It may be kept in mind that sometimes seemingly normal mucus membrane color do not rule out significant disease. Petechiae (red/ purple spots on mucus membrane) are suggestive of hemorrhages. Mucus membranes of pale white, yellowish, bluish, reddish, chocolate brown or cherry red color indicates pathological state. Pale white mucus membranes indicate anemia. Yellowish color of the mucus membranes is suggestive of jaundice, Cyanotic or muddy mucus membranes are suggestive of severe hypoxemia or decompensatory shock. Capillary refill time (CRT) reflects the perfusion of peripheral tissues. It is conducted on gums. An area of gums is pressed. On pressing the area is blanched white and turns pink again within 2 seconds when pressure is released in normal cases. Prolonged CRT (> 2 seconds) indicates compromised circulation leading to poor perfusion. It may be due to dehydration, anemia, shock, cardiac disease, hypothermia. An early

CRT (<1 second) is suggestive of hyper dynamic states as seen in cases of fever, heat stroke (hyperthermia), distributive shock or an early compensatory stage of hypovolemic shock.

5. *Systemic Body Examination (from Head to Toe)*: Systematic body examination begins with the examination of head and neck (including ears, eyes, nose, mouth), integument, thoracic limbs , thorax, abdomen, pelvic limbs and tail, external uro-genitals , perineal region, and rectum (Figure10).

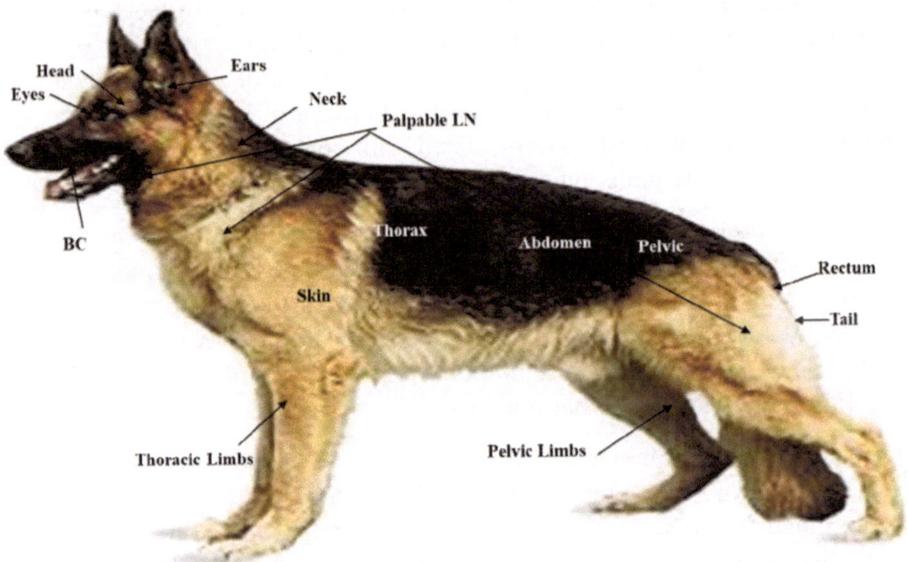

Figure 10. Diagram showing points of examination from head to toe in order of sequence.

Examination of head and neck begins with assessing the shape and symmetry of the skull followed by examination of eyes (position, movement, vision, eye lids, conjunctiva, papillary response to pen torch light, palpebral and menace response, lens position and its clarity, eye discharge or blepharospasm, color of the eye), ear (response of pinna to sound, skin of the pinna ,swelling at ear pinna, ear canal for discharge), nose (shape of external nose, symmetry, nares for the discharge and patency), buccal cavity (mucus membrane for color, moistness, petechiae/ecchymosis; gums for capillary refill time, color and integrity of palate, teeth, tonsils ; salivary mucocele- Figure11 etc.), neck (mandibular lymph nodes –Figure12 and mandibular salivary glands, flexion and extension of neck , thyroid glands, jugular vein for jugular pulse).

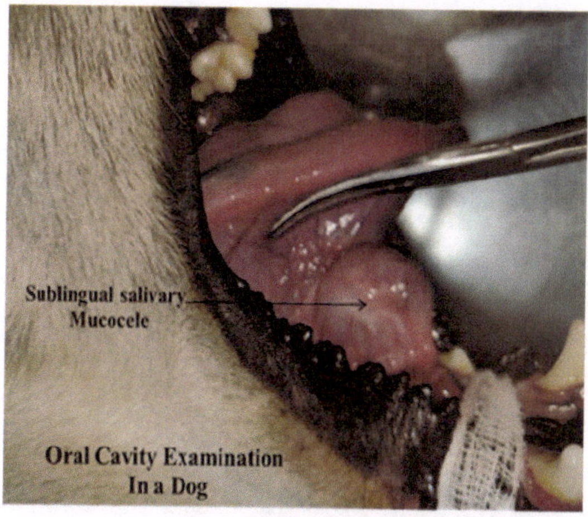

Figure 11: Showing sublingual salivary mucocele in a dog.

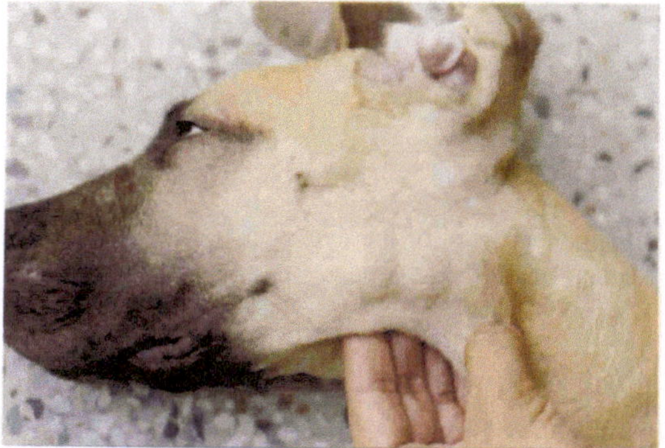

Figure 12: Showing swollen lymph node

The color of mucus membrane (Figure13) provides important information about perfusion. Mucus membrane of pink color (Figure13 A) indicates adequate perfusion of peripheral tissue and healthy state. Pale or/white mucus membrane (Figure13 B) reflects poor perfusion, loss of blood (anemia) or vasoconstriction. In cases of hypoxemia (inadequate oxygenation) mucus membrane becomes cyanotic or congested (Figure13 C).

Brick red color of the conjunctiva is suggestive of increased perfusion or vasodilation as seen in cases of fever, hyperthermia, early shock, or systemic inflammation .Yellowish (icteric) mucus membrane (Figure13D) is indicative of increased accumulation of bilirubin owing to hemolysis, hepatic diseases or biliary diseases. Petechiae on mucus membrane are suggestive of coagulation disorder such as coagulation factor deficiency, platelet disorder, or disseminated intravascular coagulation.

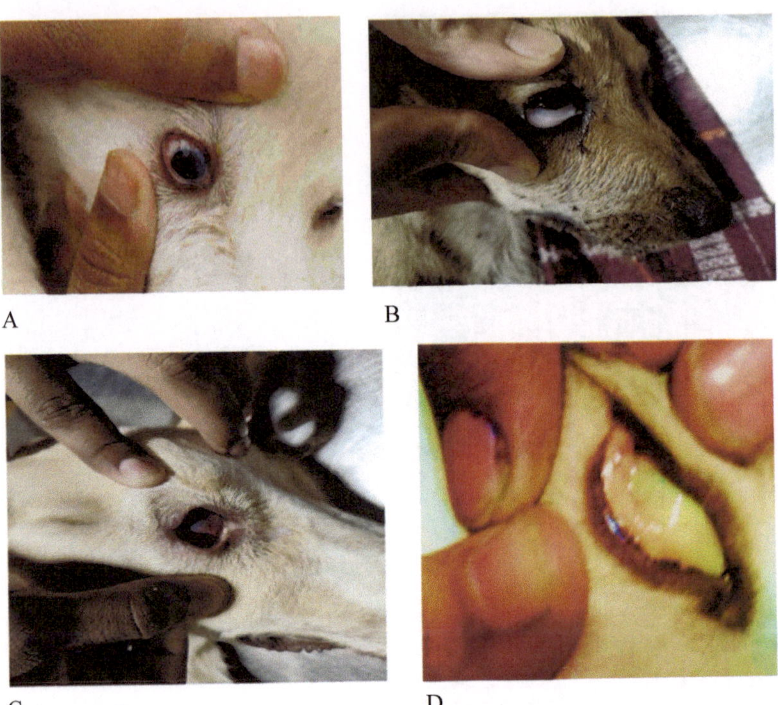

A B

C D

Figure 13: Showing different colors of mucus membrane of the eye. **A.** Normal pink. Mucus membrane. **B.** Pale or white mucus membrane. **C.** Congested mucus membrane. **D.** Icteric eye.

Jugular vein is examined for its pulsation and pressure. Jugular veins directly reflects right ventricular filling pressure during systole and diastole and right atrial pressure during systole. Jugular vein normally collapses when head is tilted up at an angle of 45^0, during inspiration or immediately after 2nd heart sound. In healthy subjects jugular veins are not distended. If distended jugular vein (Figure 14) does not collapse, it may indicate heart failure, chronic obstructive pulmonary disease, pulmonary fibrosis or ventricular filling defect due to pericardial disease. Hepatojugular reflex is a valuable adjunct in the diagnosis of congestive heart failure. Though jugular veins can be examined in standing, sitting or sternal recumbency, standing position is preferred. Hepatojugular reflex test is conducted on standing dogs and cats by compressing cranial abdomen and observing the jugular veins. Pushing up the cranial abdomen increases venous return and elevation in jugular venous pressure persists throughout the period positive pressure is applied to the abdomen. The added jugular distension or positive hepato-jugular reflex indicates right heart failure, tricuspid valve disease or pericardial disease.

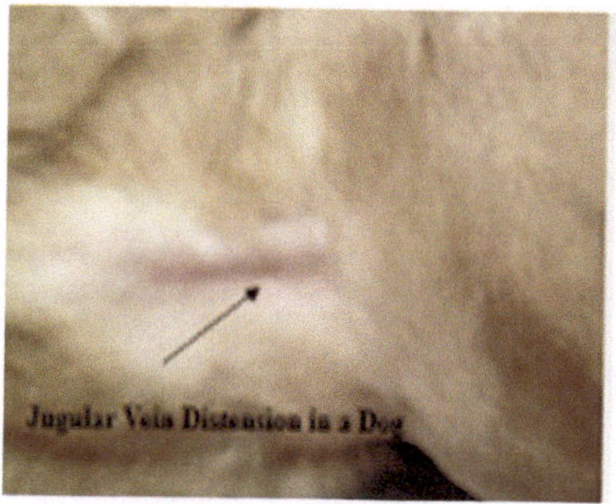

Figure 14: Showing distended jugular vein

Examination of integument is conducted by running both hands on the entire body surface .It gives an idea about the condition of the skin and hair coat. The presence of alopecia, masses (cutaneous/subcutaneous), ectoparasites (ticks - Figure 15A, fleas- Figure 15B, lice), scales , erythema (Figure15C) , petechiae (Figure15D), papules, pustules (Figure15E), ecchymosis or thickened elephant like skin (Figure15F) can be ascertained. Skin turgor can also be assessed. Entire chain of mammary glands (Figure15C) can be palpated for detecting any mass (15 G) if any.

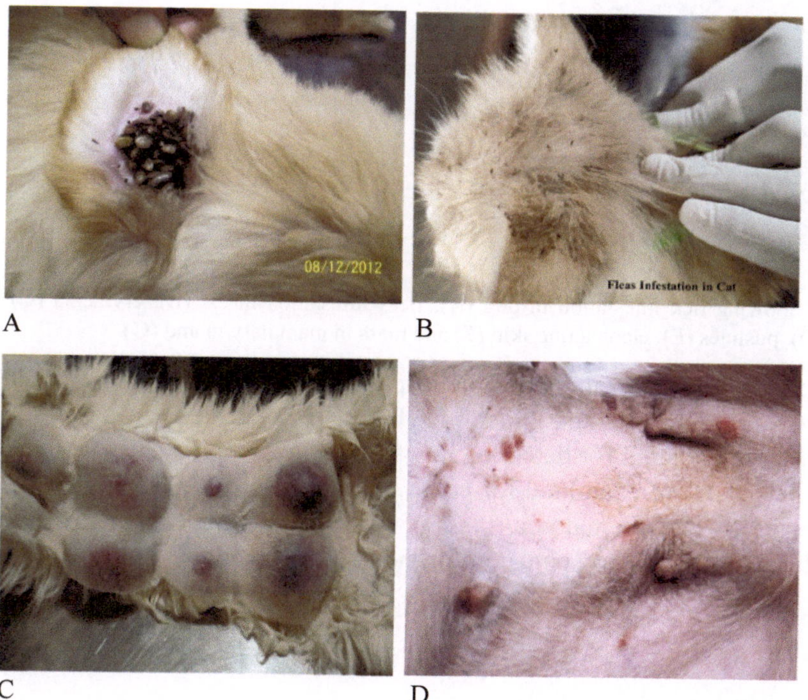

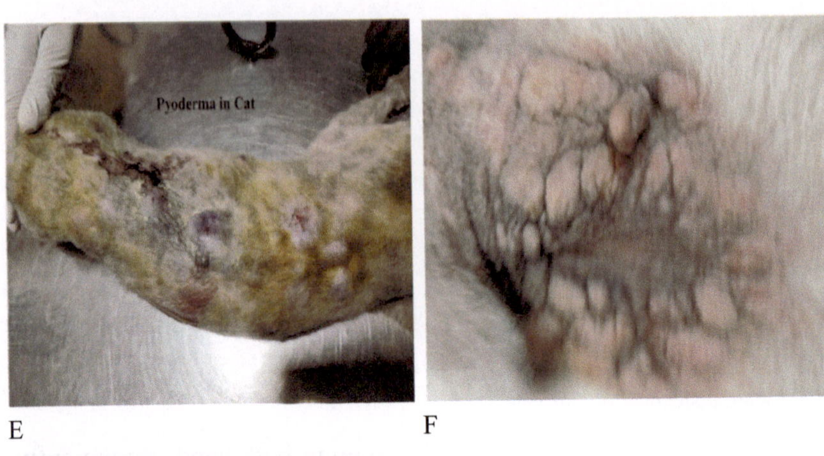

E F

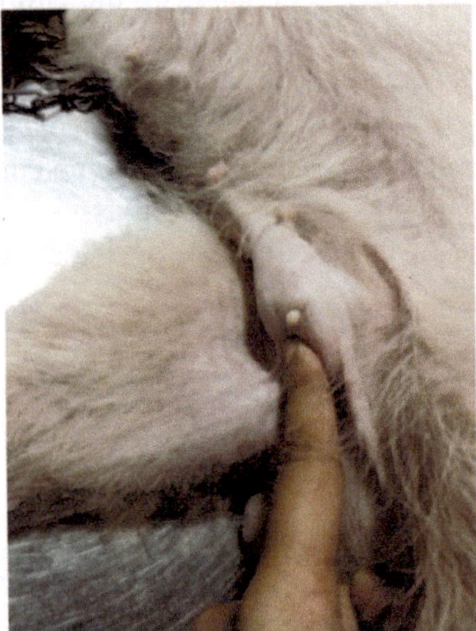

G

Figure 15: Showing tick infestation in dog **(A)**, fleas infestation in cat **(B)**, erythema **(C)**, petechiae **(D)**, pustules **(E)**, elephantine skin **(F)** and mass in mammary glamd **(G)**.

Both thoracic limbs are examined from scapula to toe. Any abnormality such as pain, no weight bearing and knuckling (Figure16 A) is noted, if any. Joint and muscles are palpated for detecting any swelling, pain and heat. Foot pad, nails and nail beds are examined for color, symmetry, erosion, foreign body, mass, interdigital cyst/ hematoma/ mass (Figure 16B) /wound or dermatitis. Prescapular lymph nodes are palpated for their size and shape.

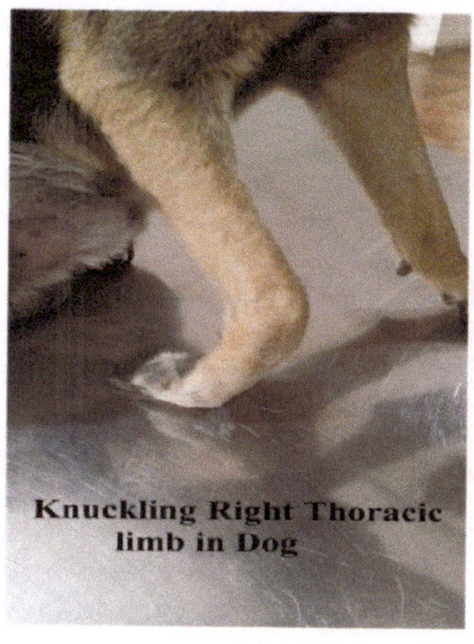

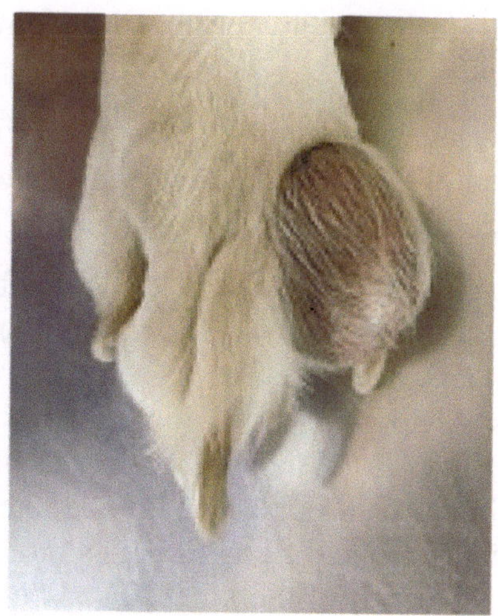

A B

Figure 16: Examination of thoracic limb in dogs. **A**. Knuckling of right thoracic limb. **B.** Mass in interdigital space

Thoracic cage is examined for its symmetry, integrity of the ribs, spinal hyperesthesia or deformity. Thorax is auscultated for assessing lung sounds ;and heart rate and rhythm. It can assist in detecting inspiratory or expiratory dyspnea, vesicular (normal) or adventitious (abnormal sounds such as wheezes, crackles) sounds. Normal lung sounds are bronchial sounds arising from turbulent airflow generated within the normal trachea and larger airways in the lungs . Normal lung sounds are usually audible dorsal to the base of the heart. Normal inspiratory sounds are soft and low pitched whereas expiratory sounds are even softer and lower in pitch. Lung sounds may be increased or decreased. Panting increases loudness and intensity of bronchial sounds. Adventitious sounds are abnormal or pathological sounds. Adventitious lung sounds are classified as continuous or discontinuous.

Wheezes are the example of continuous adventitious sound and crackle are the example of discontinuous adventitious sounds. Crackles are associated with pulmonary edema. Wheezes are associated with bronchitis and feline asthma.

Cardiac auscultation should be done on both sides of the thorax in standing position in all valve areas. Normal heart sound is two character sound "lub and dub". While murmurs are abnormal extra sounds commonly occurring between the lub and the dub having shooshing or wooshing quality.

Murmur are caused by an increase in turbulence or change in the way the blood flows through heart. Murmurs are audible in cases of structural defect in the valves, anemia, fever, infection, dirofilariasis ,hyperthyroidism or hypertension.

Most heart murmurs are audible parasternally in cats. Auscultation of the heart and evaluation of the femoral artery pulse should be done simultaneously to detect pulse deficit.

Abdomen is palpated using light but forceful touch moving the fingers in cranial to caudal and dorsal to ventral directions. For abdominal palpation tips of the fingers are used to detect mass, if any or to evaluate the size and shape of the organs. Abdominal distension (Fig .17) or pain is also noted. In healthy dogs and cats liver is not palpable as it does not extend beyond costal margin. Kidneys are located in dorso-cranial abdomen. In dogs kidneys are fixed in retroperitoneal space and right kidney is more cranial than the left kidney. In dogs, only caudal end of the kidneys can be felt. While in cats, each kidney can be felt and palpated as kidney are more mobile. In many healthy dogs tail of the spleen can be felt on the left ventral abdominal floor. Intestines are palpated throughout the abdominal cavity. In dorsal abdomen colon can be palpated. Fecal matter in the colon may be mistaken as mass. Fully distended urinary bladder is palpable in the caudal abdomen. The inguinal lymph nodes are generally not palpable in healthy subjects.

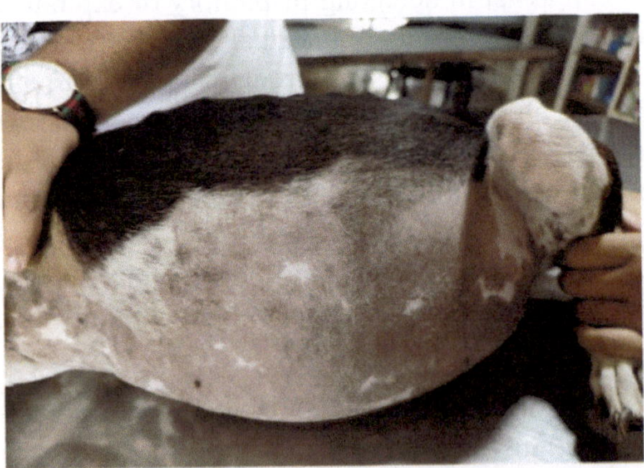

Figure 17. Showing distended abdomen in a dog due to ascites

Pelvic limbs are palpated in the manner similar to thoracic limbs. Any abnormality such as pain, limping, edema (Figure18A), knuckling (Figure18 B), if any, is noted. Joint and muscles are palpated for detecting any swelling, pain and heat. Foot pad, nails and nail beds are examined for color, symmetry, erosion, hyperkeratosis (18 C) foreign body, mass, interdigital cyst/ hematoma/ mass/wound or dermatitis. Tail is examined for its movement, hair loss and skin lesions (Figure19). Palpation of the tail can detect the presence of any tumor or swelling, if any. Lumbosacral pain can be detected by applying gentle pressure to the base of the tail. Popliteal lymph nodes (Figure 20) can be palpated behind the stifles.

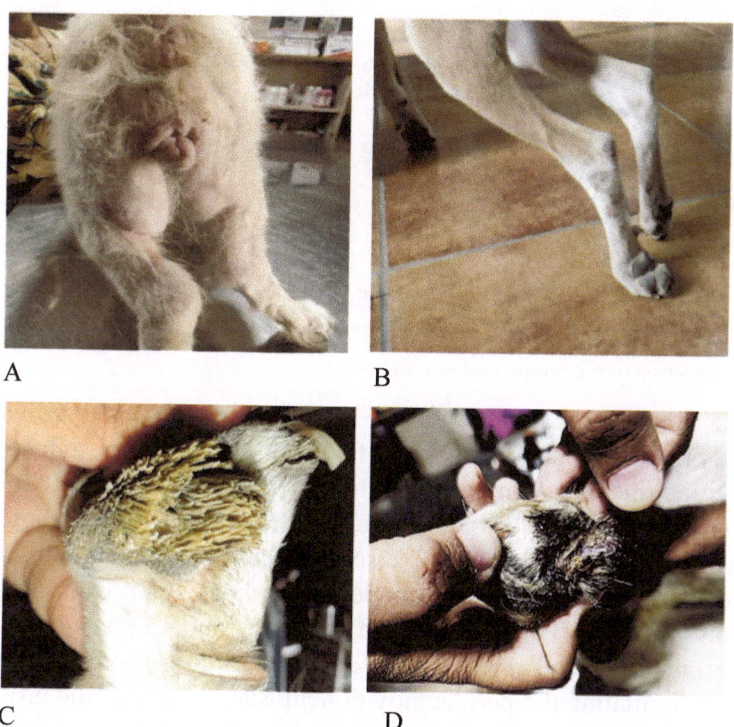

Figure 18: Showing edema **(A)**, knuckling **(B)**, hyperkeratosis frond like projections growing off **(C)** and wound **(D)** in pelvic limb of dogs.

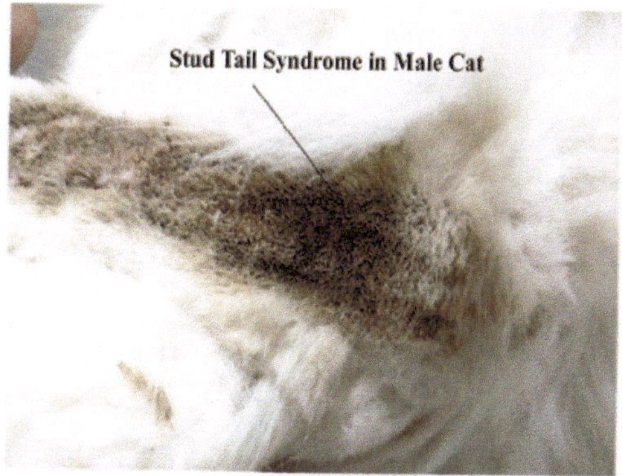

Figure 19: Showing greasy skin lesions on the dorsum of the tail.

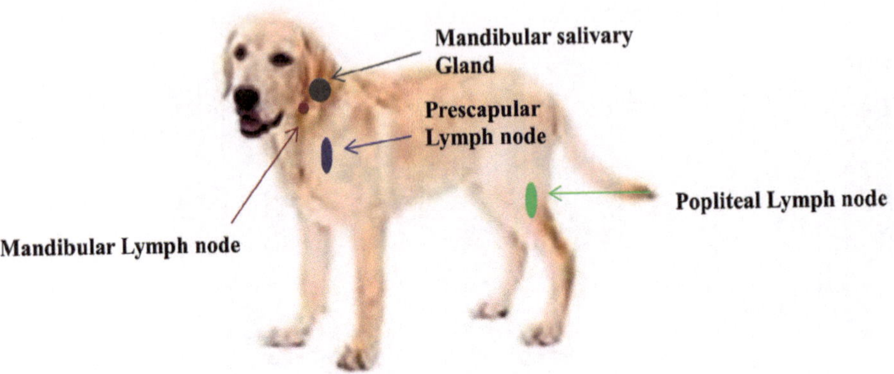

Figure 20: Showing location of the lymph nodes in the dog.

External genitalia and perineal area should also invariably be examined. Vulva (Figure21A), and prepuce should be examined for discharge, swelling, redness or any growth. Examine the symmetry of the testicles and whether both testicles have completely descended or not (Figure 21B). Any lesion (swelling, wound etc.) on testicles (Figure21C) should also be noted. Penis is exteriorized (Figure21D) and examined for venereal granuloma. Perineal area is examined for swelling , mass (Figure21E), or fistula. Integrity of caudal nerves of the tail, the prudendal nerve, spinal cord segment and associated nerve roots can be ascertained by stimulating the perineum with hemostat using a gentle prod which will cause flexion of the tail and contraction of anal sphincter.

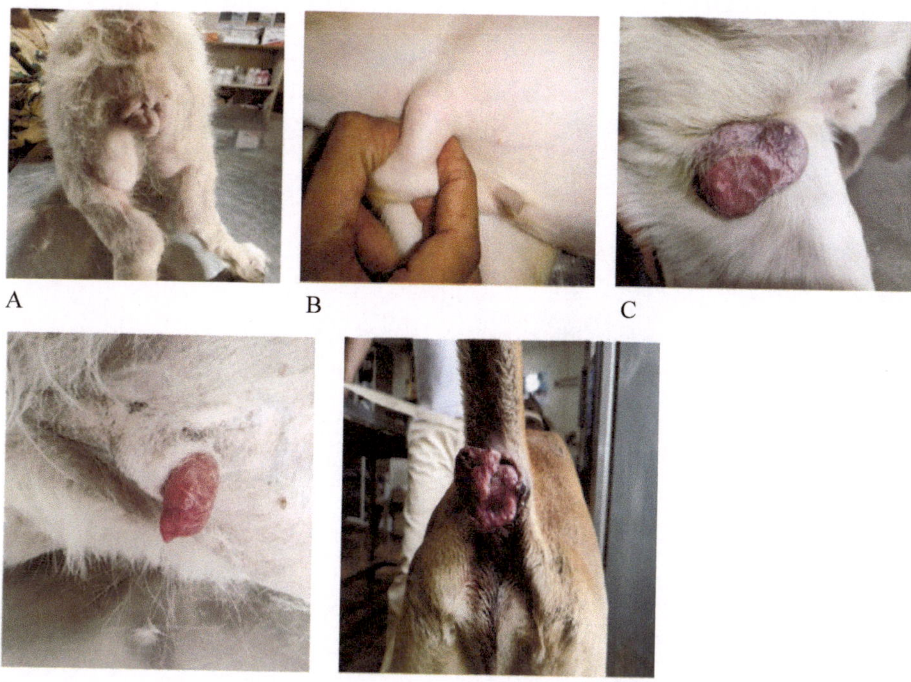

Figure 21: Showing external genitalia and perineal area. A. Normal Vulva. B. Retention of one testicle. C. Scrotal sac dermatitis. D. Normal Penis having no venereal granuloma lesions. E. Growth in perineal region.

Per rectal examination (Figure22) is conducted to evaluate rectal wall thickness, anal glands, pelvic urethra, prostates in male, and vaginal tract in females. The position of anal glands is normally at 4 and 8 –o'clock positions. During per rectal examination, feces can also be examined for color and consistency.

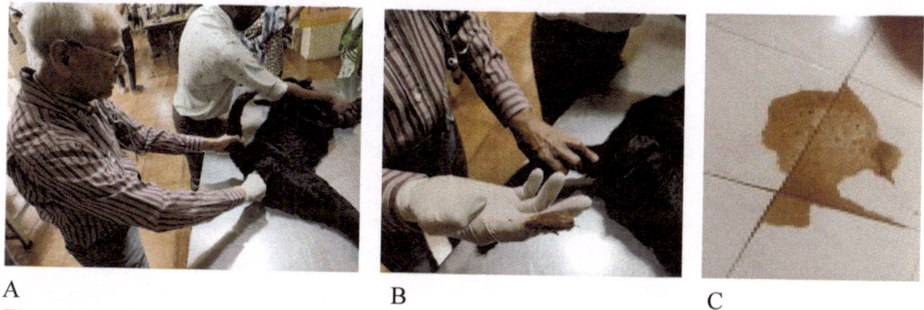

Figure 22. Showing per rectal examination in dog. A. Per rectal examination in process. B. Examination of feces for color and consistency. C. Blood mixed watery feces.

2

Centesis

Centesis is a surgical puncture or perforation into body cavity or structure usually done to aspirate fluid, air or tissue. The medical purpose of puncturing body cavities is not only to obtain fluid sample for diagnostic purpose but also to remove excessive fluid for therapeutic purpose for alleviating the respiratory distress owing to excessive fluid accumulation in peritoneal cavity, pleural cavity or pericardial sac. This procedure is usually done to get fluid from abdominal cavity, thoracic cavity, pericardial sac or joint capsule and is aptly known as abdominocentesis, thoracentesis, pericardiocentesis or arthrocentesis respectively.

Abdominocentesis /Peritoneocentesis/Abdominal Paracentesis

Abdominocentesis, peritoneocentesis, abdominal paracentesis or paracentesis abdominis is a technique of percutaneous collection of peritoneal fluid using a syringe and needle or small catheter. It is simple, rapid and safe technique routinely used for the collection of fluid from peritoneal cavity in canine and feline practice. The procedure can be performed on an outpatient basis.

Indications of the Technique

1. The technique is indicated for diagnosis purpose when there is unexplained presence of free abdominal fluid (Figure 23). Peritoneal fluid is collected for cytological, microbial and /or biochemical analysis to ascertain etiological diagnosis.

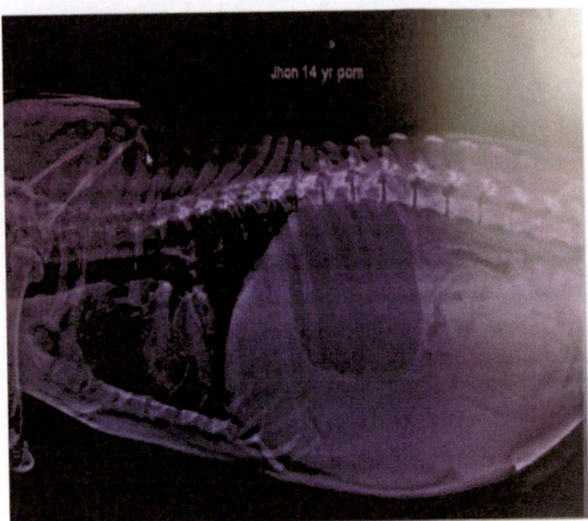

Figure 23: Radiograph of a dog showing free fluid in the peritoneum (ascites).

2. In cats the technique is recommended to obtain peritoneal fluid for the diagnosis of feline infectious peritonitis.
3. The technique is also indicated to remove considerable amount of peritoneal fluid to ease respiratory embarrassment.

Contraindications of the Technique

Abdominoentesis is contraindicated in the following conditions:

1. Organomegaly (hepatic , splenic)
2. Coagulopathy
3. Uterine diseases.
4. Injuries restricting positioning of the pet.
5. Skin infection at the site.

Precautions

1. Before performing abdominocentesis using blind puncture, it is necessary to weigh gain and risk analysis specially when a large vascular abdominal mass, enlarged vascular organ, pyometra or coagulopathy is suspected. In such cases it is always advisable to opt for ultrasound guided fluid collection rather than blind abdominocentesis.
2. Plain abdominal radiograph should be obtained before resorting to abdominocentesis to identify hollow organ rupture or peritoneal perforation if any.

Equipments

- Muzzle or Mask
- Clippers, shaving material, sterile absorbent cotton and antiseptic material for scrubbing.
- Sterile Gloves
- Sterile 21-22 gauge, 1 1/2-inch needles
- Sterile syringe
- Sterile gauze
- EDTA tube
- Plain tube /Sterile vial for culture

Procedure

Dogs/cats are placed in lateral recumbency so that large area of the ventral abdomen is available for site selection. Proper restrain is applied. Usually no sedation is needed in most of the cases. Linea alba (down to the ventral abdomen between left and right hind limbs) usually around 4-5 cm caudal to xiphoid (Figure 24) is the most preferred site for conducting paracentesis abdominis because of less vasculature in the this area and minimum chance of contamination .This area is swabbed with alcohol. Linea alba is carefully pierced using a sterile needle (21 - 22 gauge) and a syringe (5ml /10 ml) through the skin, subcutaneous tissue, and abdominal wall and into peritoneal cavity. As soon as needle pierces peritoneal cavity fluid drops appear in the syringe .The fluid is then drawn slowly. Two to three ml content of the syringe is transferred into a well labelled vials or vacutainer tubes containing EDTA for cell count , protein analysis and cytological evaluation. Other 2- 3 ml fluid portion should be transferred in to a sterile vacutainer tube or vial without anticoagulant for bacterial culture and biochemical (bilirubin, cholesterol, triglyceride, creatinine etc.) analysis.

Complications of the Technique

Trauma to internal organs is an complication of the blind paracentesis abdominis. Injuries restricting positioning of the pet and skin infection at the site are the contraindications of the procedure.

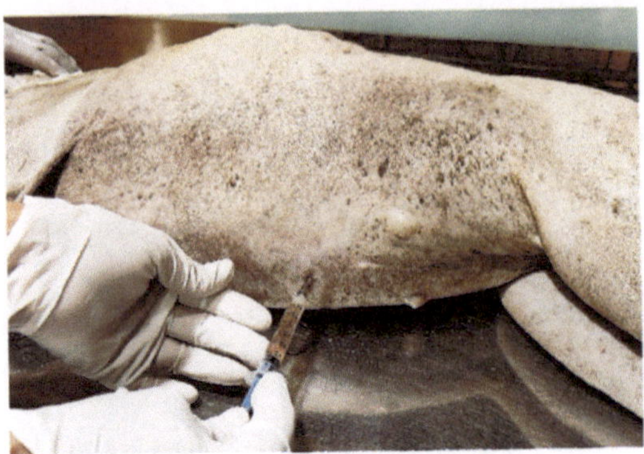

Figure 24: Showing site and collection of peritoneal effusion in a dog with peritoneal effusion (ascites).

Thoracentesis

Thoracenteseis is a minimal invasive procedure to collect or to remove pleural fluid from the pleural cavity using a syringe and needle or a small catheter. It is also a life saving technique for severely dyspnoeic pets with pleural space disease.

Indications of the Technique

The technique has both diagnostic and therapeutic purpose.

1. The technique is indicated for diagnostic purpose in cases of pleural effusion (Figure25) requiring differentiation between chylothorax, hemothorax and pyothorax. The collected aspirate is used for cultural, microscopic, biochemical and cytological examinations

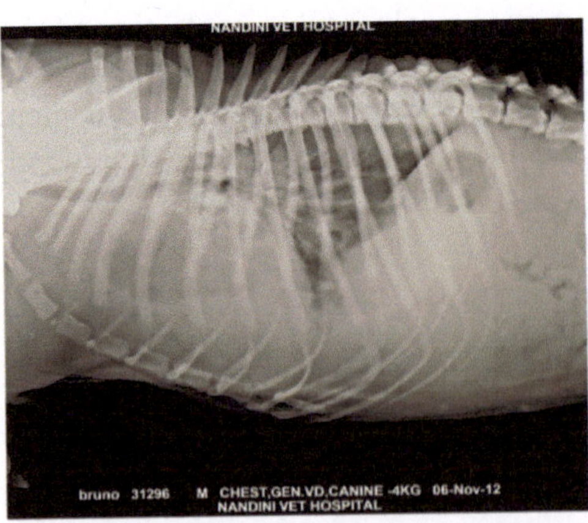

Figure 25: Right lateral radiograph of a dog showing pleural effusion.

2. The technique is indicated for therapeutic purpose also in pets to relieve respiratory distress associated with pleural effusion or pneumothorax.

Risk Associated with the Procedure

1. Excessive bleeding may occur.
2. If proper aseptic procedure is not adopted there are chances of introducing infection.
3. There may be respiratory distress.
4. Pneumothorax or collapsed lung is another risk associated with thoracentesis.

Equipments

1. Sterile gloves .
2. Lidocaine or xylocaine 2% for local anesthesia.
3. Needle or catheter of suitable length to penetrate the chest wall.
4. 3- or 4-way stopcock.
5. IV extension tubing.
6. 50 ml syringe.
7. EDTA tube and plain top tubs for sample collection.
8. Basin to hold evacuated effusion.

Procedure

Thoracentesis is often performed on both sides of the chest. The dog /cat is placed in sternal recumbency. Sedation is usually not required in dogs. One attendant/ owner is needed to restrain the pet while the procedure is being performed. Another person is required to assist with the procedure. Some cats may require short acting or reversible sedative. Ketamine hydrochloride (11-15 mg/kg) with diazepam (0.22-0.55 mg/kg IV) is suitable for performing thoracentesis in cats.

Site is prepared by clipping both sides of the chest (5th to the 11th intercostal space right from costochondral junction below to about 65% of the way up the chest wall). When pneumothorax is suspected the thorax is clipped dorsally up to the spine. The whole site is scrubbed with alcohol to sterilize the site. 7th to 8th intercostals space on the left thorax and 6th to 7th intercostals space on the right thorax are located and xylocaine (2%) is infiltrated in the area at the puncture site. Ultrasound can be used to ascertain the site. The needle or catheter is attached to the extension tubing. It is attached to the stopcock and in turn attached to the syringe. Strict aseptic condition is to be maintained throughout the procedure. The needle is inserted perpendicular to skin through chest (thoracic) wall in the chosen site (7th or 8th intercostals space on left side or 6th to 7th intercostals space on the right side) on the cranial side of the rib (so as to avoid puncturing intercostals vessels) and is advanced slowly . The needle is positioned ventrally in case effusion is suspected or it may be placed dorsally if pneumothorax is suspected. As the needle is being advanced into the chest (thorax), the assistant handling the syringe applies a little suction to allow immediate aspiration of any effusion so as to avoid introducing pneumothorax during the procedure. Once fluid (in case of pleural effusion) or air (in case of pneumothorax start flowing in to extension tubing, the needle should be manually secured by the veterinarian and assistant holding the syringe should gently aspirate the effusion in to the syringe until fluid stops flowing and negative pressure is felt. In case of pneumothorax, evacuation is continued until negative pressure is felt again. Excessive suction is avoided. Once it is ascertained that no more fluid/ air is available, needle withdrawal is started. The procedure is repeated on the other side of the thorax using new sterile supplies.

Thoracic radiographs and /or ultrasonography should be resorted to assess the amount of residual fluid.

Post Procedural Considerations

A chest X-ray or ultrasound may be considered after the procedure to detect any complication of the thoracentesis.

Pericardiocentesis

Pericardiocentesis is a sterile minimal invasive procedure to collect or remove excess fluid from the pericardial sac. It is a lifesaving procedure to relieve life threatening pericardial tamponade associated with severe pericardial effusion.

Indications of the Technique

The technique has both diagnostic and therapeutic purpose.

1. The technique is performed to collect pericardial fluid from cases of pericardial effusion (Figure26) for diagnostic purpose. The collected fluid is used for cytological and cultural examinations to detect different causes of pericardial effusions.

2. The technique is indicated as an emergency procedure for therapeutic purpose in pets to relieve cardiac tamponade associated with severe pericardial effusion.

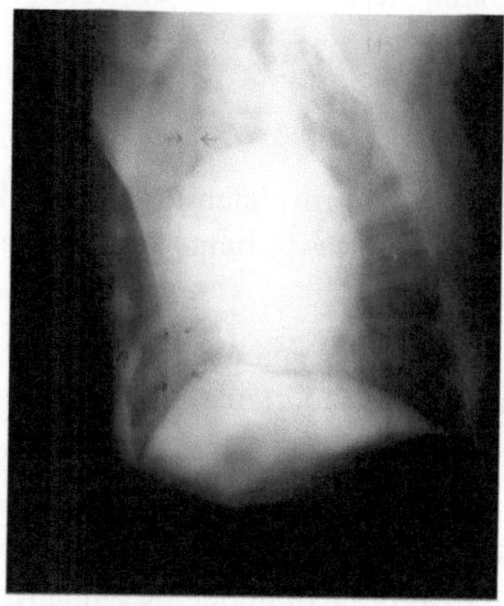

Figure 26: Dorso-ventral radiograph of a dog showing pericardial effusion.

3. In cats, pericardiocentesis is recommended in cases of feline infectious peritonitis, congenital or acquired myocardial disease, pericardial or heart base neoplasia, septic pericarditis or hemorrhages due to warfarin toxicity.

Potential Risks of the Technique

1. Laceration of myocardium or coronary arteries.
2. Incomplete drainage from the pericardial sac.
3. Recurrence of effusions.

Equipment

1. Clippers and disinfectant.
2. Sterile gloves and drapes.
3. Electrocardiograph.
4. Ultrasound.
5. Large intravenous catheter (10-14 gauge , 10-15 cm for large dogs; 16-18 gauge , 4-6 cm for small dogs and cats).
6. 3- or 4-way stopcock

7. IV extension tubing.
8. 50 ml syringe.
9. Sample collection containers (EDTA, plain, sterile for culture).
10. Lidocaine or xylocaine (2%)

Procedure

Pericardiocentesis is a sterile procedure performed in lateral or sternal recumbency from right side of the thorax to avoid injuries to lungs and carotid arteries.

1. Sedation with butorphanol (0.2 mg/kg IV) with or without acepromazine (0.005 mg/kg IV) or midazolam (0.2 mg/kg) can facilitate the procedure.
2. Constant monitoring with continuous electrocardiography is needed during the procedure. If severe ventricular tachycardia develops, it should be treated with lidocaine (2.0mg/kg IV).The technique of pericardiocentesis can be performed either as blind or under the guidance of an ultrasound.
3. Blind pericardiocentesis is done between 3rd and 5th intercostals space on right side of the thorax. While ultrasound guided pericardiocentesis is done on the right side at a place of largest diameter of the effusion.
4. The skin of the area over the 2nd to 8th intercostals space on the right side from the sternum to mid thorax is shaved, cleaned with alcohol or an antiseptic. Xylocaine (2%) is infiltrated in the skin, intercostals muscle and pleura of the site. The area around the site is draped with sterile drape.
5. The intravenous catheter, extension set with three-way stopcock and syringe are prepared in a sterile manner. If catheter is large, a small stab incision can be made to facilitate the insertion of the cannula.
6. Puncture should be done in the middle of the intercostal space so that trauma to intercostal vessel is avoided.
7. The catheter is slowly inserted perpendicular to the skin through the skin, intercostals muscle, pleura and pericardial sac. Piercing of pericardial sac is indicated by the loss of resistance and the appearance of the fluid at the catheter hub. Pericardial fluid can be aspirated.
8. In case of concurrent pleural effusion, straw colored fluid appears when needle/ catheter pierces pleural space. The catheter is advanced a little

further and stylet is removed and connection to collecting system is made.

9. If scratching or tapping sensation is felt, it indicates that the catheter is in contact with the heart warranting immediate slight retraction.
10. Samples are collected in plain tube, EDTA tube and in sterile tube.
11. When no more fluid is aspirated or needed, the catheter is retrieved.

Complications

Usually pericardiocentesis is a relatively safe procedure. Nevertheless, ventricular premature beats/ ventricular tachycardia is the most common complication owing to myocardial injury by the catheter. Coronary artery laceration, ventricular puncture, pneumothorax or hemorrhages are the other less common complications that may occur during the process of pericardiocentesis. Pericardial effusion reoccurs commonly even after removal of excess pericardial fluid. Recurrence of pericardial effusion is within hours in case of ruptured hemangiosarcoma or may be after weeks in case of idiopathic pericardial effusion.

Limitations

Expertise and procedural experience of the operator is of great value.

Arthrocentesis

It is a minimum invasive surgical procedure usually done to get synovial fluid from within a joint capsule for both diagnostic as well as therapeutic purposes.

Indications

1. Evaluation of synovial fluid for understanding etiology of arthritis and to differentiate between septic and inflammatory arthritis. Analysis of synovial fluid is also desired in disorders with persisting or fluctuating fever of unknown etiology, shifting lameness or general malaise with arthralgia.
2. Arthrocentesis is also indicated to inject contrast media in the joint for radiography.
3. The procedure is also done to aspirate large and painful joint effusions to provide relief from pain.
4. The technique can also be used to administer intrasynovial drugs.

Selection criteria for Arthrocentesis

1. Joints showing radiographic evidence of affection.
2. Visible enlarged joint.
3. Joints with overlying skin having lesion or infection are not suitable candidate for arthrocentesis.

Advantages of the Technique

1. Allows quick assessment of color and viscosity.
2. Multiple joints can be sampled.
3. Usually no sedation is needed.

Disadvantages of the Technique

1. Small yield of the synovial fluid.
2. Analgesia may be required in some joints.
3. Repeat multiple sampling from same joint may yield confusing result owing to iatrogenic bleeding.

Risk Factors

Though arthrocentesis is a minor surgical procedure conducted in outpatient department or in small operation theater, it is always associated with a risk of injuring blood vessels, nerves and tendons.

Contra-indications

1. Overlying cellulitis.
2. Coagulopathy.
3. Bleeding disorders.
4. Acute fracture.
5. Adjacent osteomyelitis.

Equipment

1. Antiseptic solutions such as betadine, chlorhexadine.
2. Skin marking pen.
3. Sterile gloves, gauge, syringes (3 ml).

4. Sterile needles (22 gauge 1-1.5 inch suitable for stifle; 22-25 gauge 0.75 inch long needles suitable for other joints; Large dogs 22 gauge 1.0 to 1.5 inch long; small dogs 25 gauge 0.75 inch long). For hip joint, a spinal needle of 3 inch and 20 or 22 gauge is more appropriate. For shoulder joint, spinal needle of 1.5 inch and 22 gauge is preferred. Always prefer smallest gauge needle to pierce joint space of joints other than stifle without causing trauma.
5. Specimen tubes (for cell count, culture and sensitivity, crystal analysis for gout).

Procedure

1. Arthrocentesis is usually performed in lateral recumbency. The joint is flexed and extended so that joint space is palpable.
2. Sometimes sedation/general anesthesia may be needed. Sedation can be achieved with dexmedetomidine (0.5 mg/ml @0.1 ml/40 lb) and butorphanol (10 mg/ml @ 0.1 ml/40 lb) as recommended by Degner (2014).
3. An area of approximately 4 to 6 cm^2 over the joint (from where synovial fluid is to be collected) is clipped/ shaved and aseptically prepared by applying antiseptic solution.

(a) **Shoulder joint:** Dog is placed in lateral recumbency with the shoulder joint in a neutral position. Shoulder joint can be approached from lateral or cranial sites. In lateral approach the dog is placed in lateral recumbency with fore limb parallel to the table and shoulder joint partially flexed. Needle is inserted just cranial to glenohumeral ligament and slightly (about 0.5 cm) distal to the acromion process of the scapula in a lateral-to-medial direction (Figure27). In cranial approach the dog is placed in lateral recumbency with partially flexed shoulder joint. Needle is inserted medial and proximal to the lateral aspect of greater tubercle of the humerus, ventral and lateral to the supraglenoid tubercle of the scapula and advanced slightly dorsal along intertubercular groove (ventral to the acromion of the scapula).

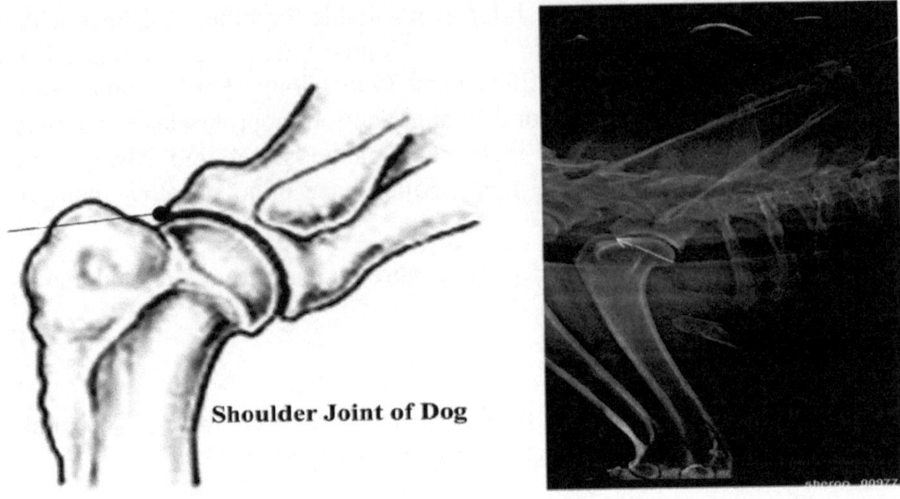

Figure 27: Shoulder Joint of the dog. **A.** Drawing of shoulder joint of the dog. Black circle indicates the target joint space. **B.** Radiograph of shoulder joint of the dog showing target joint space (marked by white arrow).

(b) Elbow: Dog is placed in lateral recumbency with affected elbow downward. The joint is flexed slightly and caudal aspect of the joint is palpated. The joint space is between humeral condyle and olecranon (Figure 28). The needle is inserted into the skin just caudal to lateral aspect of epicondyl of the humerus just above the dorsal edge of olecranon. The joint space is small. Care should be taken so that needle remain parallel to the dorsal edge of the olecranon.

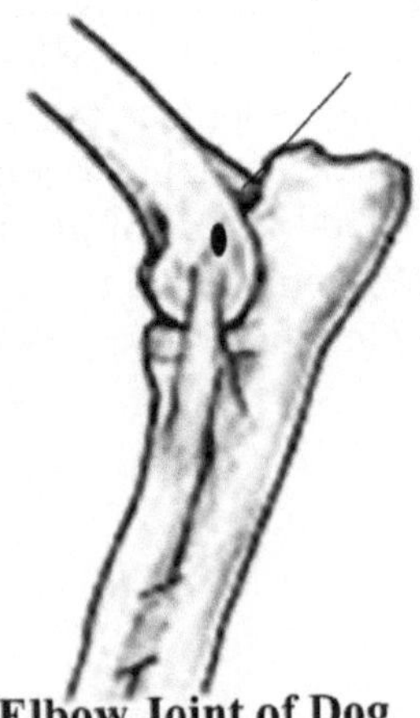

Figure 28: Drawing of elbow joint of the dog. Black circle indicates the target joint space.

(c) **Carpus:** Dog is placed in lateral recumbency with the affected limb upward. The radio carpal joint is the largest carpal joints to aspirate from the cranial side. Flexing the carpus joint by 45° facilitates needle entry. The dorsal surface of the radiocarpal joint is palpated to detect joint space and the needle is inserted perpendicular to the dorsal surface of the joint. Joint space is very superficial. Therefore deep insertion is to be avoided. Intercarpal joint can be aspirated in similar manner but the joint space is very narrow.

(d) **Hip:** The dog is placed in lateral recumbency with the hip upward in slight abduction and external rotation. Spinal needle (3inch long) of 22 or 20-gauge is inserted just dorsal to the greater trochanter, and is moved in a lateral-to-medial direction. Another approach is a ventral approach. In which needle is inserted just caudal to the pectineus muscle over the hip joint (Figure29) and is directed at a 45° angle in a craniodorsal direction. Some resistance may be felt as the needle is passed through the ventral joint. Ultrasound guidance is helpful but not essential.

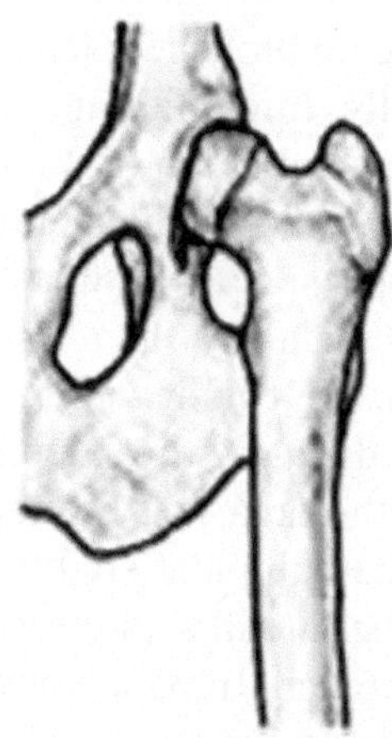

Figure 29: Drawing of hip joint of the dog

(e) **Stifle:** Stifle joint is shown in the drawing and x-ray (Figure30) to understand the location. The dog is placed in dorsal recumbency with the stifle flexed. The needle is inserted slightly lateral to patellar tendon (half way between distal patella and tibial tuberosity. The needle is directed caudally and slightly medially (towards the opposite condyle). The joint space is deeper.

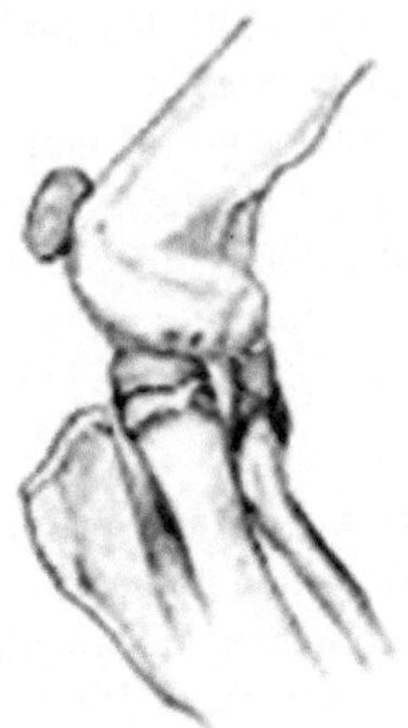

A

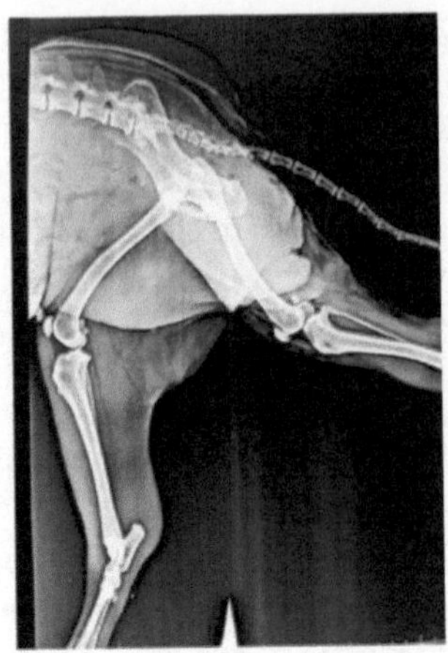

B

Figure 30: Drawing **(A)** and X-ray of stifle joint **(B)** of dog

(f) **Tarsus:** The dog is placed in lateral recumbency with the limb in question on top. The lateral aspect of the joint is preferred as it gives better yield of the fluid. The tarsus joint can be approached from cranio-laterally (anterior), laterally, or caudo-laterally. In cranio-lateral approach, the joint is flexed and extended to facilitate palpation of joint space between the distal tibia and tibiotarsal bone on the craniolateral surface of the joint. Needle is inserted into the joint space just distal to the end of the tibia. The needle is now directed caudally at an angle of 45^0 into the tibiotarsal joint. In lateral approach, joint is flexed and extended so as to facilitate palpation of the joint distal to the lateral malleolus of the fibula. The needle is inserted in the area just caudal to malleolus of the fibula directing the needle tip medially and slightly cranially. Care should be taken to avoid piercing the lateral saphenous vein in this area. Another option is caudolateral approach. In which, the joint is flexed and extended to palpate the joint space between distal tibia and trochlea of the talus. The distal tibia is on the medial side, fibula is on the lateral side and the talus is on the caudal side of the joint space. The joint is moderately flexed and the needle is inserted slightly caudal and medial to the lateral malleolus of the fibula. Needle fitted with syringe is used. Needle is firmly gripped with finger and thumb, directed downwards, is inserted through the skin into the joint space. In case, the bone is felt while advancing the needle, withdraw it slightly, and re-direct. Aspiration is done gently. Usually a small amount of fluid is retrievable unless the joint is grossly distended, Excessive forceful aspiration may lead to contamination of the fluid with blood. Aspiration (negative pressure) is to be stopped prior to withdrawing the needle from the joint space.

Precautions

1. The process of collection of synovial fluid influences the results of analysis and interpretation.
2. Inadvertent rupture of blood vessel may cause hemodilution of synovial fluid leading to alteration of total nucleated cell count and differential cell count.

Reference

Degner, A.D. (2014). Arthrocentesis in dogs. Clinician's Brief (August, 2014): 69-74.

3

Catheterization and Pneumocystography

Catheterization is done for both diagnostic as well as therapeutic purpose. As a diagnostic technique it is employed to collect urine samples, prostatic wash and suction biopsy. As a therapeutic technique it is used for the treatment of urine retention, obstruction and for monitoring urine output. Pneumocystography is a contrast radiography. It is being employed to distinguish the urinary bladder from other organs and to visualize the details of the bladder.

Catheterization

An appropriate catheter needs to be selected as per the requirement (purpose of catheterization and duration of catheterization). A soft, silicone flexible catheter is appropriate for indwelling purpose. Whereas a rigid catheter is more desirable to unblock a small calculi and collecting samples for diagnostic purpose. Small size catheters are best in order to minimize urethral trauma.

Equipments Required

Equipment requirement depends on the purpose of catheterization. Whether catheterization is required for indwelling, unblocking the calculi, collection of urine sample, or need of anesthesia/sedation. Generally clippers, non-irritating diluted antiseptic solution, gauge swab, syringes for flushing, lubricant, sterile urinary catheter of appropriate size and type, sterile close collection tubes/vials, gloves (sterile, disposable), equipment for sedation/anesthesia, Elizabethan collar (to prevent patient interference) are needed. If the catheter is to be indwelled, sterile saline, sterile needle and suture material, needle holder, thumb forceps and scissors may also be needed. The size of the catheters for dogs (Figure31) varies from 5 FG (1.65 mm) to 28 FG (9.24 mm). One F is equivalent to 0.33mm. Length of the catheters also varies. Generally 500 mm effective length catheters are more commonly available for dogs.

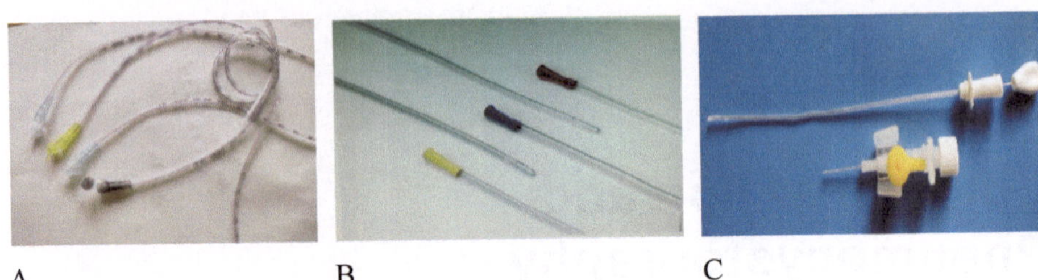

A B C

Figure 31: Showing catheters for dogs **(A and B)** and tom cat **(C)**

Patient Preparation

Hairs around prepuce/ vulva are to be trimmed, cleaned and a non-irritating antiseptic solution is applied around the area to minimize the chance of contamination and ascending infection of urinary tract. The inside of the prepuce / vulva is flushed with diluted non-irritating antiseptic solution.

Procedure of Placement of the Catheter

The dog/cat is properly restrained and placed in lateral recumbency. The size of the catheter is measured from bladder neck to prepuce. Os penis is grasped and prepuce is retracted caudally to expose the glans by an assistant. The lubricated catheter is inserted into the urethra through glans penis (Figure 32). Once the catheter reaches at the level of os penis, the grip on the penis is relaxed to facilitate further insertion of the catheter into the urinary bladder. With the insertion of the catheter in to the urinary bladder, flowing of the urine begins out from the hub of the catheter. If the catheter is required to be indwelled, the Foley balloon is inflated with 0.9 % sterile saline and catheter is withdrawn slowly until balloon sits in the bladder neck.

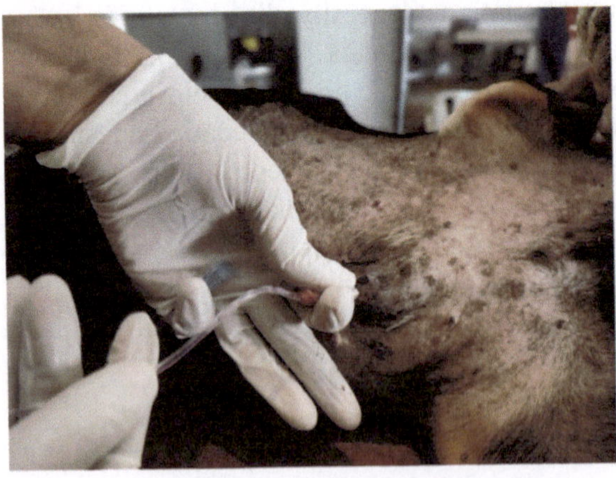

Figure 32: Showing catheterization in a male dog

The technique of placement of catheter in male cats (Figure33) is almost similar to male dogs except sedation /anesthesia may be required and the size and length of the catheter is different. The prepuce is pushed cranially with the help of thumb and index finger to expose the glans penis.

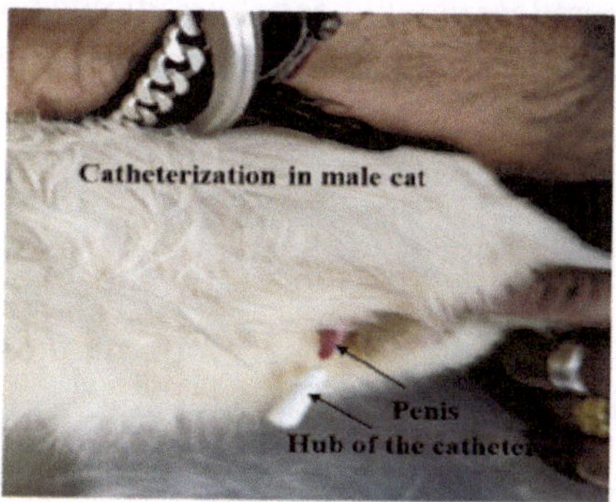

Figure 33: Showing placement of catheter in a male cat.

The placement of catheter in bitches is a little more complex. The bitch is placed in dorsal recumbency with hind limbs extended cranially or in sternal recumbency with hind limbs hanging from the table. The site is prepared as detailed above. In females the catheter is measured from the neck of the bladder to vulva. For direct visualization of urethral orifice, vaginal scope can be used. The lubricated catheter is inserted into urethral orifice with the slit directed ventrally. The catheter is moved forward until it reaches urinary bladder and urine emerges from the hub of the catheter. In blind approach external urethral orifice is palpated around 2.5 cm from the vulva along the ventral aspect of the vestibule and the catheter tip is inserted into the urethral orifice. Rest procedure is the same as in direct visualization using vaginal scope.

The technique of placement of catheter in queens (female cat) is almost similar except sedation /anesthesia may be required and the size and length of the catheter is different.

Potential Adverse Effects

- Urinary tract trauma and inflammation are potential adverse effect. It usually resolves without complications.
- Urinary tract infection is another potential adverse effect. It requires urine culture and sensitivity to control urinary tract infection.
- Perforation of urethra or urinary bladder may also occur. Diagnostic imaging is required to locate the perforation and surgical correction.

Pneumocystography

Pneumocystography is the technique of introducing the air into the urinary bladder through a urethral catheter .It is the contrast radiography. The air being radiolucent, it creates a contrast between urinary bladder and its wall. The urinary bladder borders remain radiopaque and its cavity becomes radiolucent due to air. With pneumocystography, the bladder is distinctly identified and separated from adjacent viscera.

Indications

- For visualization of extrinsic or intrinsic filling defects.
- The technique is useful in detecting cystitis, bladder wall rupture, bladder neoplasm, and calculi in urinary bladder and urethra.
- Though, the technique is inexpensive and frequently employed to determine position and integrity of the urinary bladder or to demonstrate the presence of bladder calculi, neoplasm and cystitis in dogs, it is potentially dangerous in cats as fatalities caused by air embolism have been reported. Cystitis in cats is associated with enlarged/exposed blood capillaries causing absorption of air. The absorbed air in capillaries is transported to heart and is trapped in the right ventricle obstructing the blood flow to the lungs. This risk is increased if the cat in lateral recumbency is overinflated. To minimize the risk, cats should be placed in left lateral recumbency during the procedure and over inflation of air should be avoided.

Procedure

- The technique is simple.
- A twenty four hours fast and administration of laxative and enema may result in better visualization.
- The pet may be tranquilized or anesthetized to prevent struggling.
- The pet is placed in lateral recumbency or ventrodorsal position.
- Urethral catheter is inserted as detailed above in catheterization technique.
- Urine is evacuated.
- In case of hematuria, the bladder is flushed with sterile solution of saline or sterile water to remove blood clots.
- Air is then introduced into the urinary bladder through the catheter using the sterile syringe (Figure34) with or without a three way stopcock.

There is no prescribed amount of air to be introduced. Volume of the air to be introduced is to be assessed on the basis of animal's size and its approximate bladder volume.

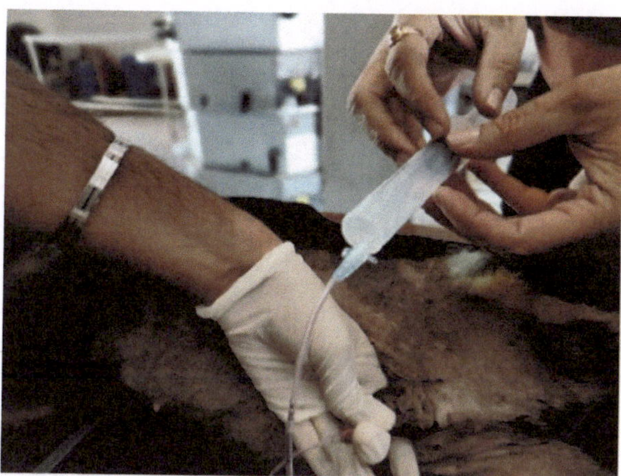

Figure 34: Showing the process of pneumocystography in a dog. The air is being pushed into the urinary bladder through inserted catheter and syringe.

- Then the radiograph (Figure35) is taken immediately to visualize the bladder.

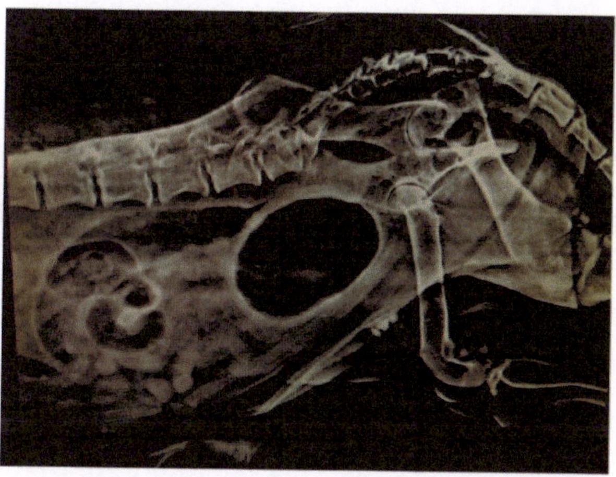

Figure 35: Showing a radiograph taken immediately just after introduction of air into the urinary bladder. An air filled urinary bladder with white regular margin of the wall and dark contents is visible in the radiograph. There is no growth or calculi in the bladder.

4

Pulse Oximetry

It is an easy, non-invasive, bed side technique for continuous monitoring the saturation of oxygen bound to hemoglobin (SpO2). The technique was invented by Dr. Takuo Aoyagi in 1974 to measure oxygen saturation in the blood. During recent years it has shown great utility in patient care. The oxygen saturation of hemoglobin provides a measure of cardio-respiratory functioning. Pulse oximeters generally used in humans are not appropriate for the use in dogs and cats as these are designed to apply on fingers and programmed with the oxygen hemoglobin dissociation curve for humans.

Indications

Pulse oximetry is an important standard technique of patient care in cases of heart failure, respiratory failure, multiple organ failure, critical care, emergency, accident and during anesthesia.

Basic Principle of Oximetry

The principle of oximetry is based on two technologies viz. Infrared spectroscopy and pulse plethysmography. Infrared spectroscopy detects the absorption of light by the tissues at two different wave lengths (visual red 660 nm wave length and infra red spectrum 940 nm wave length). Light absorption by hemoglobin at these wavelength differs depending on the level of oxygen saturation of the hemoglobin. Oxygenated hemoglobin absorbs more infrared light as compared to deoxygenated hemoglobin. The amount of light absorbed at each wave length is measured by photodetector, and the amount of oxyhemoglobin and deoxyhemoglobin in the absorbed light are calculated by microprocessor and finally displayed on the monitor.

Pulse plethysmography records the change in light absorption due to the pulsatile variation in volume of arteries and the transformation into a pulse waveform. Oximeters using this technique display oxygen saturation, heart rate and a plethysmographic trace. The variations in absorption of light are depending on variation in the amount of blood flowing underneath the probe, concentration of the erythrocytes, local blood velocity and the distance between the light source and the detector.

Oximeter

Pulse oximeter (Figure36) has two light emitting diodes (LEDs) emitting red (660 nm) and infrared (905-950nm) light and a photosensor positioned opposite the LED –the transmittance probe. There are two types of oximeters available in the market such as reflection pulse type or transmission pulse type. In former case LEDs (light emitting diodes) transmitted light is reflected back to the photodetector placed at the same side of the probe. While in later case, LEDs transmit light through tissue to the photodetector placed at the opposite side of the probe. Oximeters commonly used in animals are of transmission pulse type.

Ear lobe transmission probes used in humans can be used in dogs and cats. Whereas finger transmission probes are not very useful in animals.

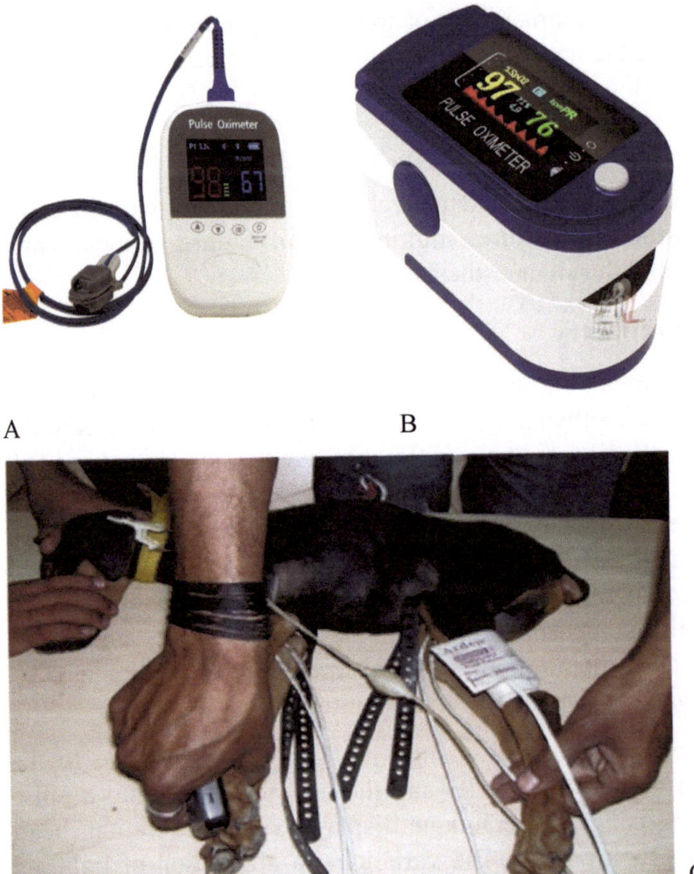

Figure 36: Pulse oximeters. **A.** For the use in dogs and cats. **B.** Fingertip oximeter being used commonly in humans. **C.** Multipara monitor used in dogs for measuring oxygen level, blood pressure and heart indices.

New Generation Pulse Oximeter

- They use different signal extraction technologies.
- Nellcor OxyMax System- It is based on resistor calibration technique.
- Masimo Pulse Oximeter System- It uses signal extraction technology based on red and infrared photoplethysmographic signals and also employs other techniques such as radiofrequency and light-shielded optical sensors, digital signal processing and adaptive filtration to analyze SpO_2.

Functions of Pulse Oximetry

- Calculates the percentage of level of oxyhemoglobin and reduced hemoglobin in the arterial blood.
- It provides continuous detection of pulsatile arterial blood in the tissue bed (probe is usually attached to tongue, ear pinna, lip or interdigital space).
- It also provides information about pulse rate.

Factors Affecting the Function of the Pulse Oximeter

- Body movements such as shivering .tremors, seizures.
- Fluorescent light during the procedure.
- Peripheral blood flow changes due to hypotension, vasoconstriction, or hypovolemia.
- Bradycardia, tachycardia and cardiac arrhythmias.
- Anemia (packed cell volume <10%) causes underestimation of the true hemoglobin saturation.
- Electrical disturbances.
- Increased levels of blood carboxyhemoglobin and /or methemoglobin.
- Dark pigmentation.
- Pulse oximeter is of no use during cardiopulmonary resuscitation because of poor pulsatile flow.

Limitations of using Pulse Oximeter in Clinical Settings

- Decreased peripheral perfusion.
- Probe positioning.

- Calibration assumption.
- It cannot identify hypoventilation in patients breathing an enriched oxygen mixture.
- It cannot identify mild to moderate degree of lung dysfunction in patient breathing an enriched oxygen mixture.
- Optical interference.
- Signal artifact.
- In cats failure of measurement and signal quality, makes pulse oximetry a challenging task.
- There may be penumbra effect if the probe is malplaced causing a distortion in absorption resulting into erroneously low SpO2 readings (Guan *et al.,* 2009).

Sites for Probe Placement

- Tongue is usually a preferred location for probe placement in dogs and cats.
- Alternate locations in cats are lip, pinna, metacarpus and metatarsus.
- For anesthetized small animals the most commonly used sites are the tongue, lips, paws, vulva, and prepuce. Lateral edge of the tongue of the large dogs, and center of the tongue of the cats has appropriate tissue thickness.

Premedication

- Medetomidine and dexmedetomidine, are commonly used for premedication in cats.

Procedure

- Photosensor is placed on the upper side and LED on the lower side of the tongue to prevent the receiver detecting overhead artificial lighting. Placement of wet gauze between tongue and probe improves the signal quality by increasing tongue perfusion, maintaining correct alignment of LED/photosensor and shielding the photosensor from the ambient light.
- While using transmission probes, it is to be ascertained that the LED and photosensor are positioned directly opposite each other to avoid distortion of the signal.

- Once the probe is adequately placed, the readings are displaced within few seconds. It provides the reading of pulse rate and arterial blood saturation with oxygen (SpO2).

Normal Values

- Normal arterial hemoglobin oxygen saturation (SaO_2) and saturation of peripheral oxygen (SpO_2) values in healthy dogs and cats, breathing room air (FiO_2 =21%), are approximately 97%. In health reading of SpO_2should be > 95-96% at minimum.

Caution

- A display a clear plethysmographic curve and the PR reading is considered correct. In case displayed PR is wrong and/or plethysmographic curve is not displayed, the SpO_2 reading needs to be discarded.

Reference

Guan, Z., Baker, K. and Sandberg, W. S. (2009). Misalignment of disposable pulse oximeter probes results in false saturation readings that influence anaesthetic management. Anaesthesia and Analgesia 109: 1530-1533.

5

Electrocardiography

Electrocardiography-A noninvasive Technique

Electrocardiography is a non-invasive diagnostic technique routinely used to examine the electrical activity of the heart in health and diseases. It is an important tool for the clinical evaluation of the heart. The technique provides important information regarding heart rate, heart rhythm, impulse formation and its conduction. Heart size can also be assessed to some extent in humans and dogs. The process of electrocardiography leads to generation of an electrocardiogram as a consequence of depolarization and repolarization of heart muscle cells during each heartbeat. This chapter on electrocardiography is by no means a complete information to make readers expert but it aims to sensitize and make you familiar with the technique and its application so that cases with compromised cardiac function are referred timely for electrocardiographic investigation. For further knowledge readers are advised to refer the books mentioned under further readings at the end of the chapter.

Electrocardiograph (Figure37) is a machine used to examine the electrical activity of the heart and produces a visible record popularly known as an electrocardiogram (Figure38).

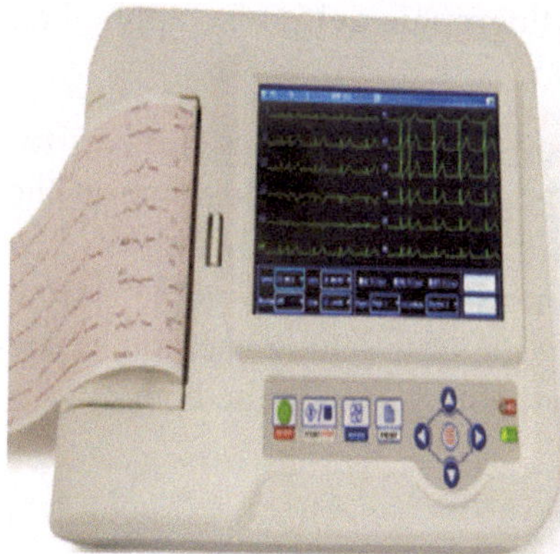

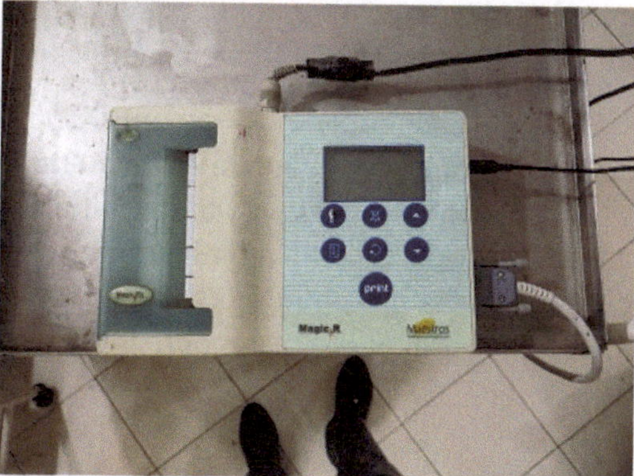

Figure 37: Six channel Electrocardiographic Machines

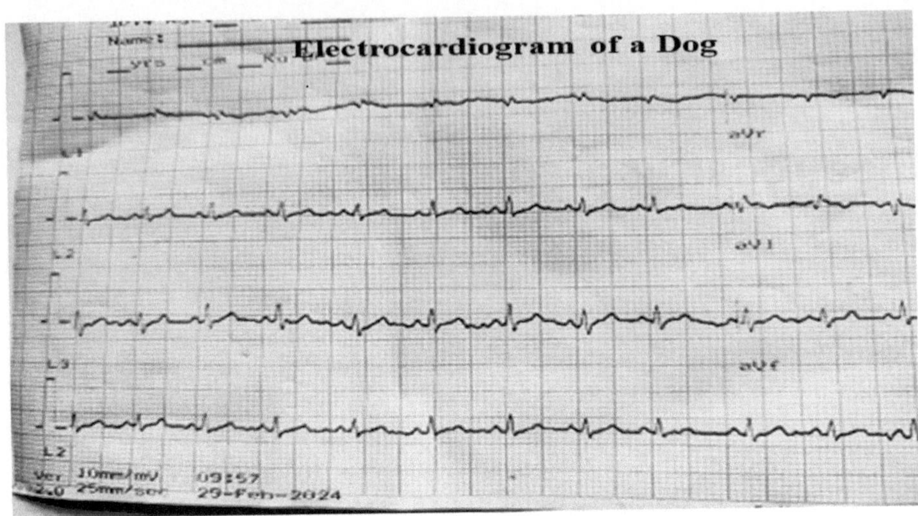

Figure 38: Electrocardiogram of a dog taken at the speed of 25 mm/second and sensitivity of 1.0 in lead I, II, III, aVR, aVL and aVF.

Dogs are restrained manually for electrocardiography and usually require no drug or medicine in most of the cases. The pets are comfortable with the presence of their owner at the electrocardiographic table while electrocardiogram is being taken. Uncooperative pets may be managed with diazepam (1 mg/Kg orally 1 hour before examination) or acetylpromazine (2 mg/Kg orally 1 hour before the examination or 0.5 mg/Kg intramuscularly or intravenously 15 min before examination) without significantly affecting the cardio-pulmonary functions.

The sites for placing the electrodes are prepared by shaving, cleaning and applying electrocardiographic gel. Electrocardiographic gel is also applied on the electrode clips to facilitate proper contact

Right lateral recumbency is the most desired position of the dogs and cats for electrocardiography (Figure39). The animal is placed in this position on the wooden table or a table covered with a foam mattress and rubber sheet. The pets are restrained by an attendant in the manner shown in the Figure39. Both left and right limbs should remain separated without touching each other and the forelimbs should be kept perpendicular to the long axis of the body.

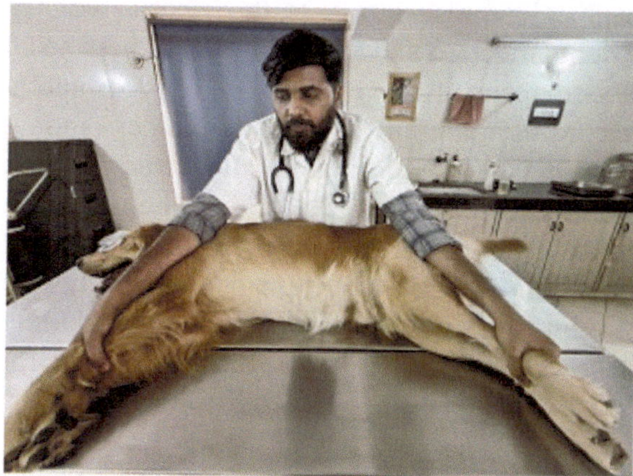

Figure 39: The dog is positioned in right lateral recumbency for electrocardiography and is restrained as shown in the picture.

Electrodes clips are applied directly on the skin of the sites (Figure40). RA and LA electrodes are attached directly on the skin proximal to the olecranon on the caudal aspect of respective fore limbs; and RL and LL electrodes are attached over patellar ligament on the anterior aspect of the respective hind limbs. V electrodes or chest electrodes are attached on skin of the chest (CV5RL at 5th right intercostal space near edge of sternum. CV6LL at 6th left intercostal space near edge of sternum, CV6LU at 6th left intercostal space at costo-chondral junction and V10 over dorsal spinous process of 7th thoracic vertebra).

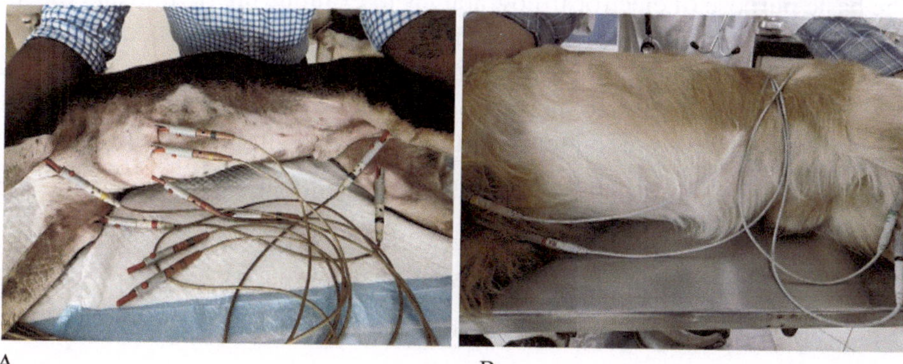

A B

Figure 40: Placement of electrodes in standard limb leads and chest leads **(A)**; and only in standard limb leads **(B)**. LA (yellow) and RA (red) electrodes are attached to the skin proximal to olecranon on the caudal aspect of the left and right fore limb respectively. LL (green) and RL (black) electrodes are attached to the skin over patellar ligament on the anterior aspect of the left and, right hind limb respectively. CV5RL electrode is attached at 5th right intercostal space near edge of sternum. CV6LL electrode is attached at 6th left intercostal space near edge of sternum, CV6LU electrode is attached at 6th left intercostal space at costo-chondral junction and V10 electrode is attached over dorsal spinous process of 7th thoracic vertebra.

An electrocardiogram is a graphical representation of the electric voltage produced during the process of depolarization and repolarization of both atrial and ventricular muscle mass plotted against time (Figure41). The information gathered in the form of an electrocardiogram in very useful in understanding the activities of the heart. An abnormal electrocardiogram may detect the side of the heart affected and abnormalities related to rate and/or rhythm of the heart. A normal electrocardiogram does not always exclude the possibility of the cardiac disease. Therefore an electrocardiogram should always be interpreted in conjunction with the result of all other examinations including detailed clinical history and observations. 'EKG'/ 'ECG' is abbreviated for electrocardiogram.

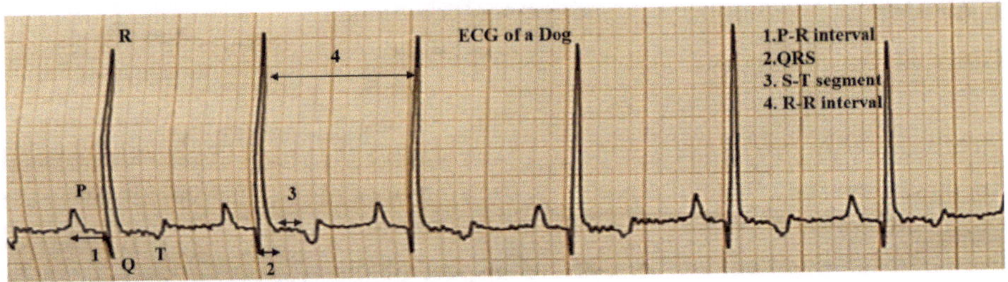

Figure 41: Electrocardiogram of a dog showing waves (marked as P,Q,R, T on the ECG) , intervals (P-R, R-R) and Segment (S-T).

Indications for Electrocardiography

The basic purpose of electrocardiography is to examine the rhythm and rate of the heart, regularity or irregularity of impulse generation and its conduction. Therefore, electrocardiography should be conducted whenever clinical examination reveals cardiac murmurs and/or slow / fast /irregular heart. The electrocardiography is of immense value in the following conditions.

1. For ascertaining the diagnosis of the disturbances of heart rate and rhythm (arrhythmias).
2. For monitoring heart during anesthesia and/or surgery.
3. For evaluating pets with respiratory distress / seizures/syncope/shock.
4. For evaluating suspected cases of cardiac diseases.
5. For evaluating heart in cases presented in emergency with hypothermia, hyperthermia, snake bites or electrocution.
6. For ascertaining cardiac status of pets with multi organ failure.
7. For evaluating heart of pets brought in emergency department.

8. For constant monitoring of heart in intensive care units.
9. For evaluating heart of geriatric patients with acute or chronic illness.
10. For evaluating heart of pets affected with ascites.
11. For Health checkup of pets engaged in sports/snuffing activities.,
12. For evaluating heart of pets with trauma/ accidents.
13. For regular cardiac monitoring of pets with heart diseases.
14. For evaluating heart of pets with electrolyte disorders or severe dehydration.
15. For regular cardiac monitoring of pets on cardiac drugs.
16. For monitoring the disease progression of the pets with heart ailments.
17. For generating database for differentiating nonspecific causes of weakness, fatigue, lethargy, syncope, collapse, seizure/epilepsy and fever.
18. For routine pre -surgical examination of the heart .
19. For routine health checkup of pets

Advantages of the Technique

1. The technique is a handy and non-invasive technique easy to use.
2. Electrocardiogram is a visual graph instantly available during the process.
3. Electrocardiogram can be read and interpreted immediately after its generation.

Limitations of the Technique

1. The technique is unsuitable for making definite diagnosis of congestive heart failure.
2. The technique is unsuitable for prognostication during anesthesia or surgery.
3. The technique is unsuitable for making definite diagnosis of the diseases of cardiac valves (mitral, aortic, pulmonic and tricuspid), endocardium, and pericardium; and wall thickness of cardiac chambers.
4. The technique is unsuitable for making diagnosis of obstructive blood flow diseases.

5. Electrocardiogram should be interpreted in conjunction with all other observations and investigations by a technically competent veterinarian as casual reading by unqualified person may lead to erroneous interpretation.

Further Readings

Varshney, J.P. (2020). Electrocardiography in Veterinary Medicine. Springer Nature, Singapore, Pte, Ltd.

Varshney,J.P.(2023). Heart Failure in Animals: Current Concepts. NIPA® GENX Electronic Resources & Solutions P. LTD. New Delhi-110 034.

Varshney,J.P., Saini, Neetu and Kumar, K.S. (2023).Electrocardiogram Made Easy for Veterinary Students and Practitioners. NIPA® GENX Electronic Resources & Solutions P. LTD. New Delhi-110 034. New Delhi-110 034.

6

Imaging Techniques

Almost all imaging techniques employed in human medicine are being followed in canine medicine but radiography and ultrasonography (abdominal and cardiac) are the most commonly used clinical diagnostic techniques. Computed tomography, magnetic resonance imaging, and nuclear techniques are also being used in the teaching establishments.

Radiography

Use of radiography (Figure 42) as a diagnostic technique is wide spread in canine and feline medicine across the world. It is considered the first step in evaluating the skeleton, thorax and abdomen. For evaluating the abdomen, radiography is considered as complimentary to sonography. Canine practice is more like pediatrics requiring assistant to control the patients (dog sand cats). No anesthesia or sedation is generally required for radiography. But if the patient has painful lesion such as fracture or luxation, suitable anesthesia / sedation should be used for making the animal cooperative during radiography for better visualization of the lesions. Multiple positions (right lateral recumbency, left lateral recumbency, dorsal recumbency, sterno-abdominal recumbency –Figure 43), depending on the direction of the X-ray beam, are used in canine and feline radiography. Anatomical planes in which radiographs generally taken are dorso-ventral , ventro-dorsal, cranial and caudal. In ventro-dorsal plane, X-ray beams enter from ventral side of the body. Contrast radiography is used to evaluate urinary tract, digestive tract and spinal cord.

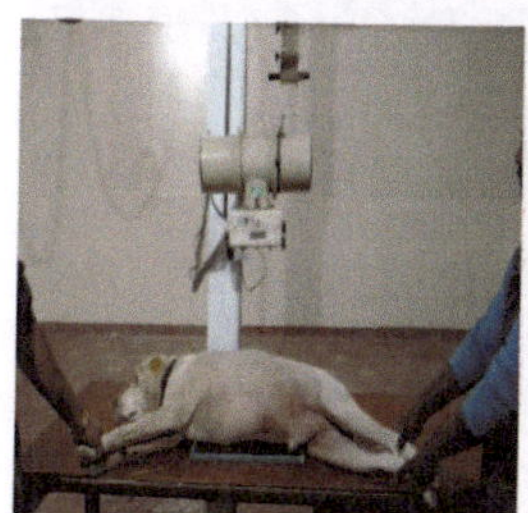
A

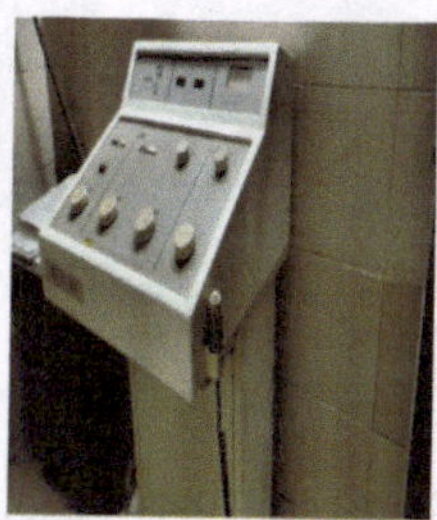
B

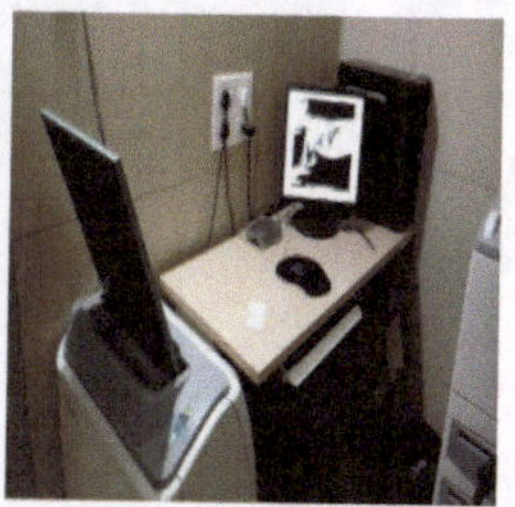
C

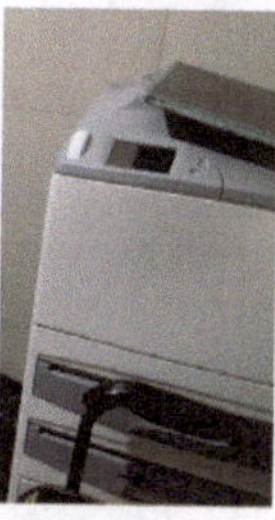
D

Figure 42: Digital Xray Machine

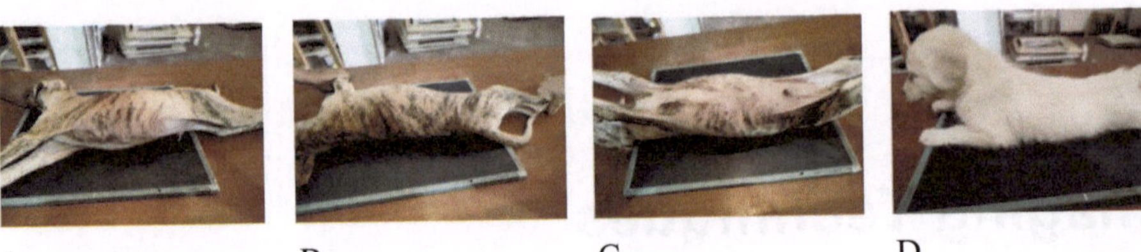

A B C D

Figure 43: Positioning of the dog for radiography. **A.** Right lateral recumbency. **B.** Left lateral recumbency. **C.** Dorsal recumbency (for VD view). **D.** Sterno-abdominal recumbency (for DV view).

Skeleton

Radiography is the best diagnostic tool to evaluate bone lesions such as bone cyst, bone tumor, hip dysplasia, patellar luxation, fracture, degenerative joint disease, osteoarthritis (Figure44), osteoporosis, and rickets ; monitoring healing process : and assessing the efficacy of treatment. Radiography is also being used for screening many congenital or hereditary osteo-articular diseases such as dysplasia (hip or elbow). Two orthogonal views should always be taken so that all bone segments are viewed.

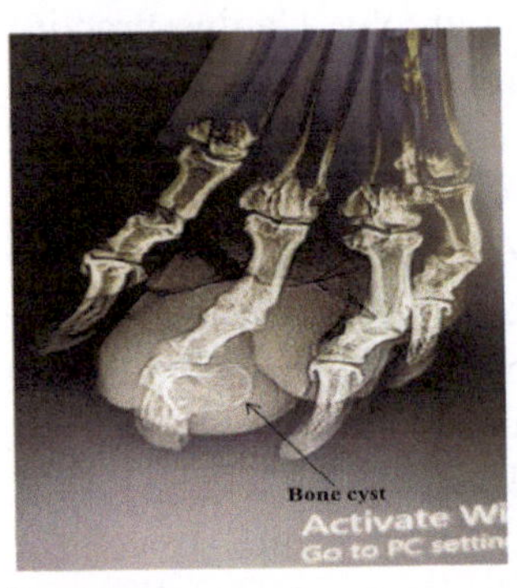

Bone cyst

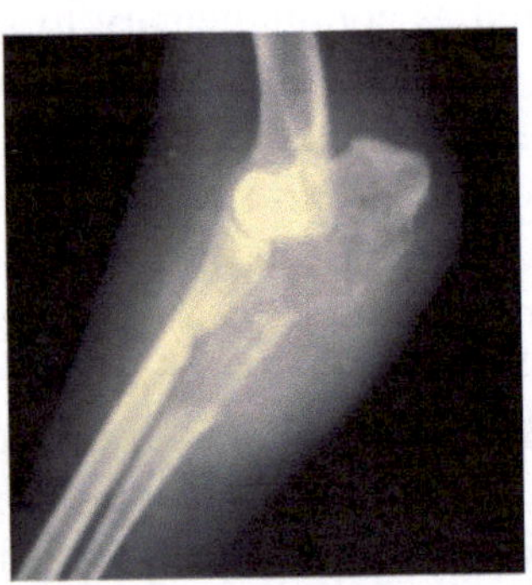

Oteolytic bone changes

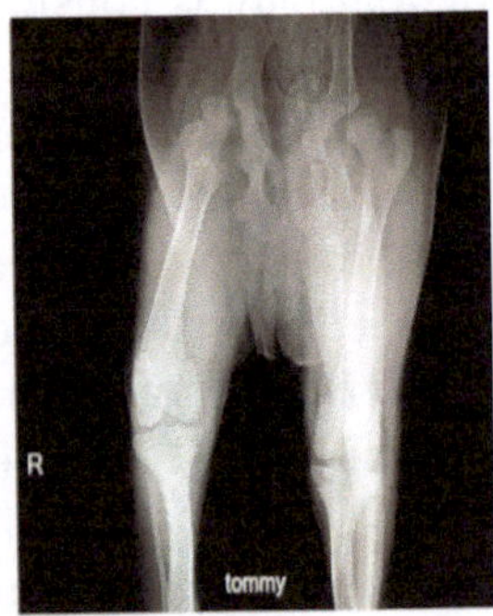

Hip dysplasia

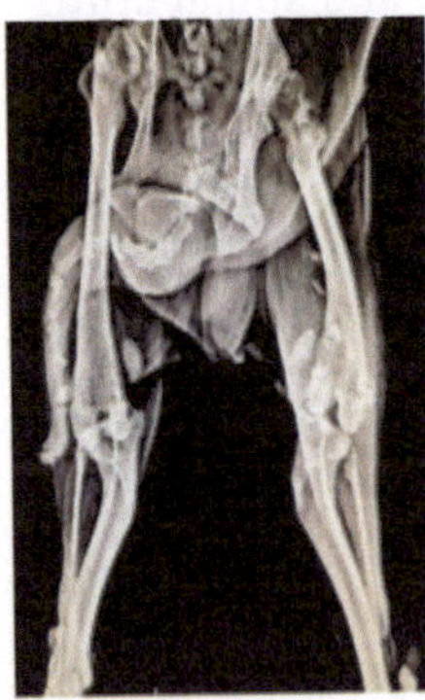

Patellar luxation

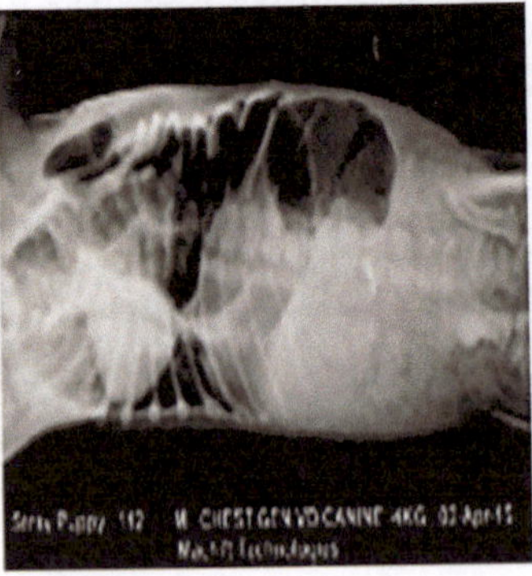

Rib fracture

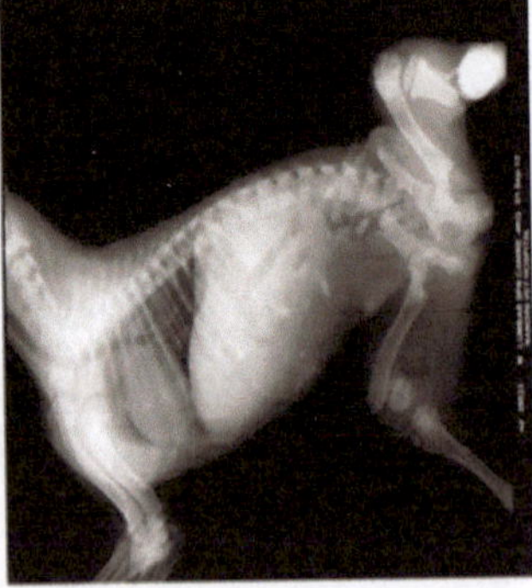

Femur fracture

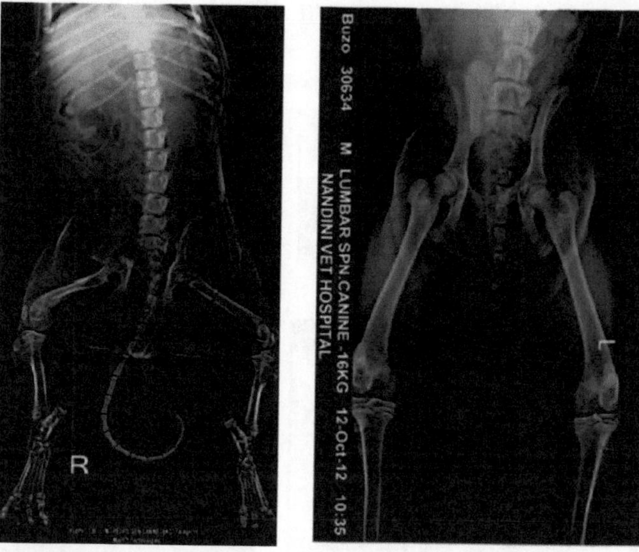

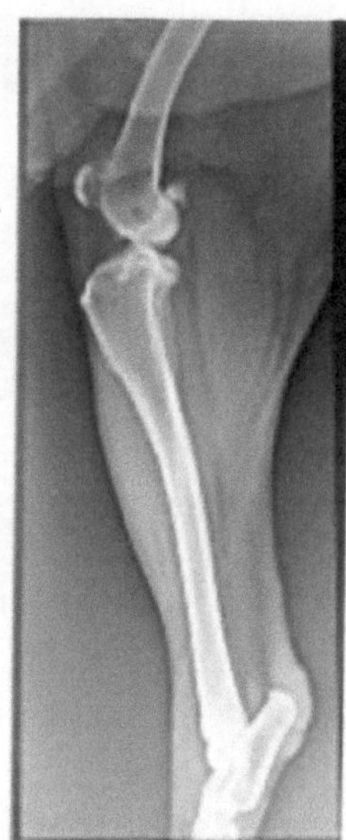

Pelvic Fracture Degenerative Joint Disease Osteoarthritis

Figure 44: Radiographs of the dogs showing different bone lesions.

The Thorax

Radiography of the thorax is a diagnostic technique of choice for assessing the thoracic organs. Air in the lungs provides good contrast to visualize thoracic organs. Thoracic radiography usually does not require any sedation or anesthesia. To avoid movements and artifacts on the image, a very short exposure (0.008 or 0.012 second) is advisable. If feasible radiograph must be taken at the end of inspiration except in cases suspected for pneumothorax. The thorax radiographs are obtained in right lateral recumbency (latero-lateral left to right to assess the esophagus, heart and left lung), left lateral recumbency (right to left to assess the heart and right lung), sterno-abdominal recumbency (dorso-ventral to assess the heart, main pulmonary vessels and dorsal portion of the lung lobes), or dorsal recumbency (ventro-dorsal to assess the ventral portion of the lung lobes, the heart, the esophagus and the mediastinum). Thoracic radiography (Figure45) in usually indicated in suspicious cases of pneumonia, congestive heart failure, taking heart dimension, esophageal stenosis, megaesophagus, tracheal stenosis, trauma and diaphragmatic hernia.

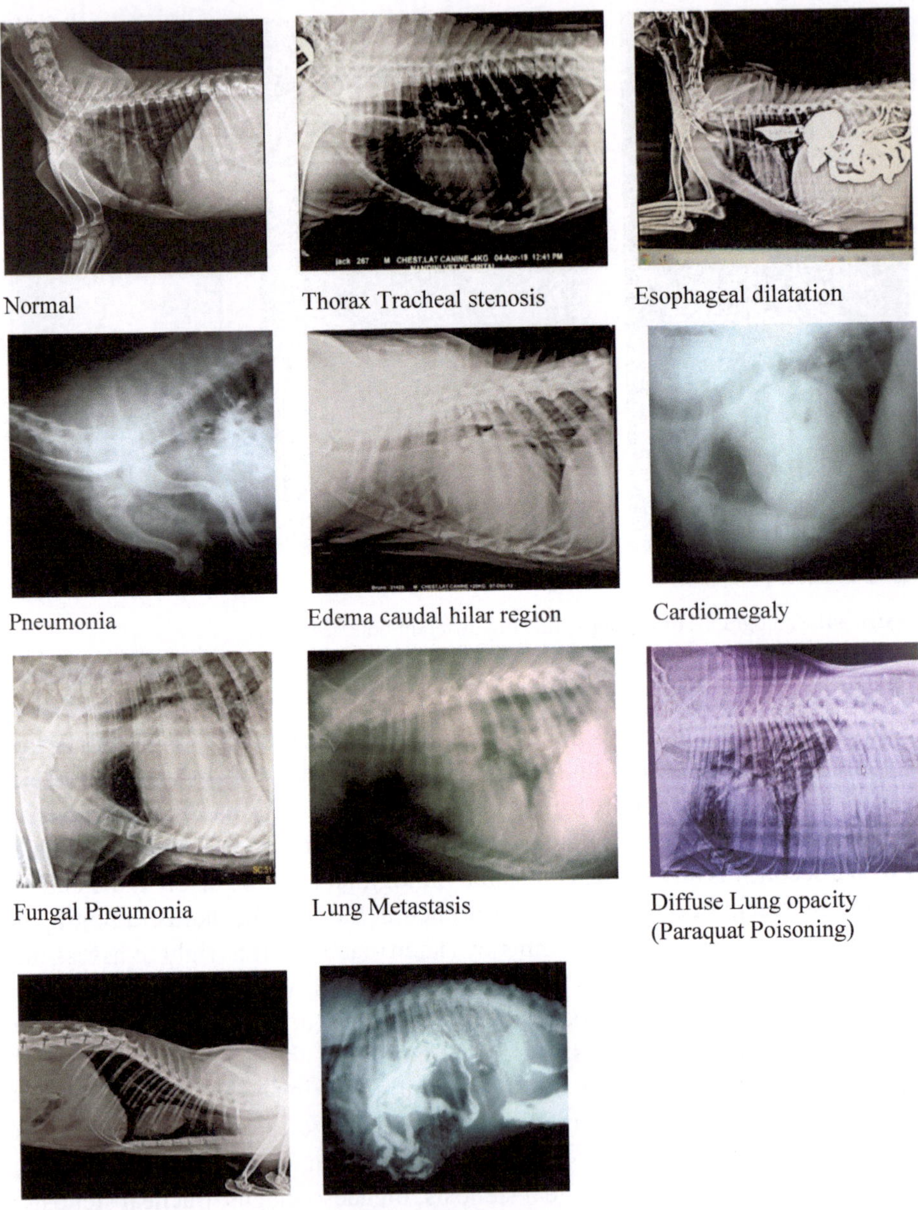

Normal

Thorax Tracheal stenosis

Esophageal dilatation

Pneumonia

Edema caudal hilar region

Cardiomegaly

Fungal Pneumonia

Lung Metastasis

Diffuse Lung opacity (Paraquat Poisoning)

Pneumothorax

Diaphragmatic hernia

Figure 45: Thoracic radiographs of dogs showing different conditions

The Abdomen

Abdominal cavity (Figure 46) broadly contains liver , gall bladder, spleen, stomach, intestines (small and large), pancreas, kidneys, ureters, urinary bladder, reproductive organs (prostates in male; ovaries, oviducts, uterus and vagina in females), adrenals and lymph nodes. Abdominal organs are made of soft tissues and therefore can be better visualized by ultrasonography. Nevertheless, abdominal radiography is also being routinely employed to have a quick overview of abdominal organs. Abdominal radiography can assists in evaluating the size, shape and position of the abdominal organs. It is a diagnostic tool of first choice when ingestion of foreign body or pronounced meteoric dilatations is suspected. It plays an important role in the diagnosis of diseases of gastrointestinal tract, urinary bladder, and other abdominal organs. Because of low contrast resolution for soft tissues, normal organs like gall bladder, pancreas, adrenal glands, ovaries, uterus and lymph nodes in healthy canine remain indistinguishable. Plain or contrast (barium meal) abdominal radiography also does not require any sedation or anesthesia. For better visualization of abdominal organs, radiographs need to be taken at the end of expiration with a less exposure time (approximately 0.016 second). In planned abdominal radiography a fasting of 12 hours or more is recommended. When colon or urinary organs are to be radiographed in a planned manner, laxative for 2-3 days and enema before the radiography provides better result. Abdominal radiography is routinely performed in latero-lateral-LL (on right or left lateral recumbency) and ventro-dorsal (VD) position. When stomach is being assessed, radiographs should be taken in both right and left lateral recumbency. For pregnancy visualization, dorso-ventral (DV) view is preferable. Evaluation of ureters and urethra needs contrast radiography. Radiography is also a valuable tool during the last period of pregnancy to ascertain the number of fetuses.

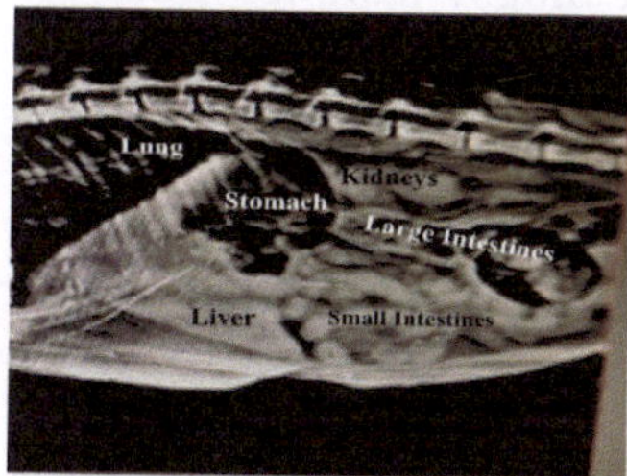

Organs of Abdominal Cavity

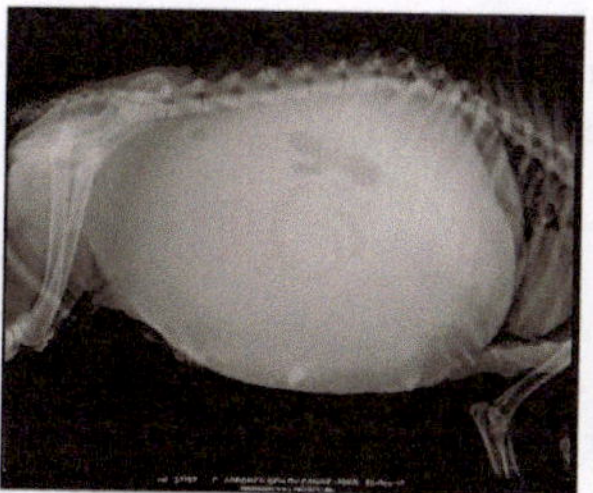
Ground-glass appearance of abdomen in ascites

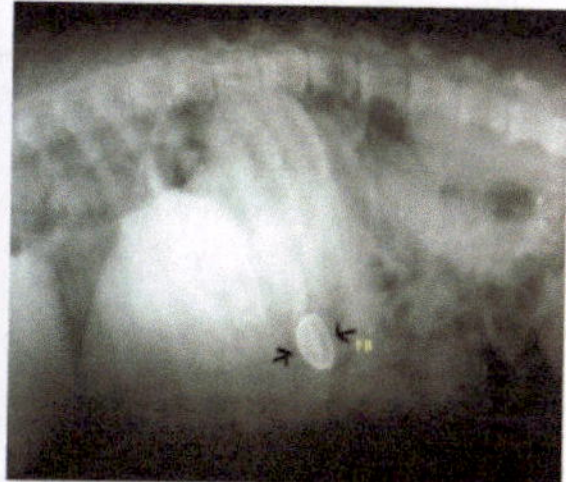
Foreign body in stomach

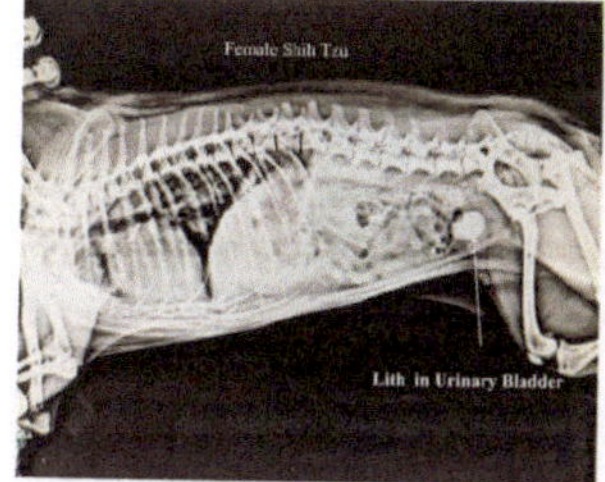

Calculi in urinary Bladder

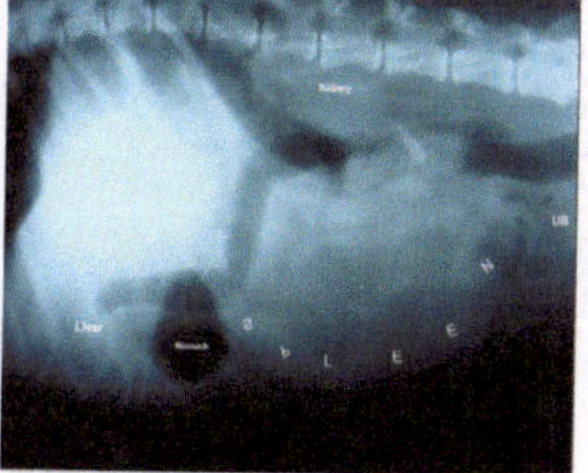
Enlarged Spleen

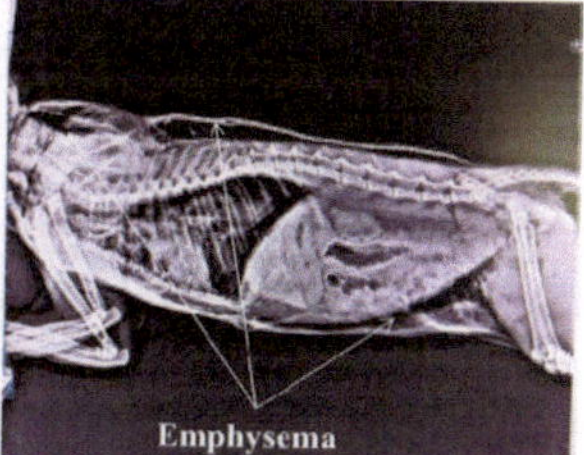

Subcutaneous emphysema

Figure 46: Abdominal radiographs of dogs showing different conditions.

Ultrasonography

The use of ultrasonography in small animal practice began in 1960s and now it has become an important diagnostic tool throughout the world. It is a non-invasive, radiation free and safe imaging technique (Figure47) to visualize internal structures of the body. The technique is highly operator dependent and needs specialized skill for correct interpretation. The application of ultrasonography generally requires no sedation/ anesthesia but needs proper preparation of the site to be imaged. Liberal application of acoustic gel on the hair free (shaved) site to be subjected to ultrasonography and on the ultrasound transducer (probe) is very much important. Other important factor is the selection of the transducer. Transducers (Figure47C) are categorized according to ultrasound frequency produced as 2.5 MHz, to 10.0MHz .Therefore, transducer is selected as per species of animal under examination and area to be scanned for generating good sonographic images. If the depth of the organ from the body surface is less (superficial organs), high frequency probe is used and when the depth of the organ to be imaged is comparatively more from the surface, low frequency probe is to be used. Ultrasonography is employed in diagnosing the diseases of the abdomen, the thorax, the musculoskeletal system and the heart. Of these, abdominal ultrasonography is the most common and important application of the ultrasound in routine canine and feline practice. It is of great utility in evaluating the liver, the gall bladder, the spleen, the kidney, the urinary bladder, the prostate, the uterus, the intestines, lymph nodes and endocrines. The technique is also used to collect biopsy samples from the internal organs. The technique of sample collection under the guidance of ultrasound is known as ultrasound guided biopsy technique.

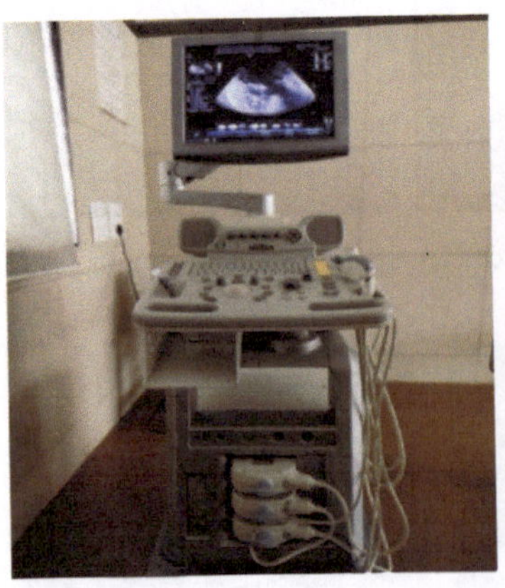

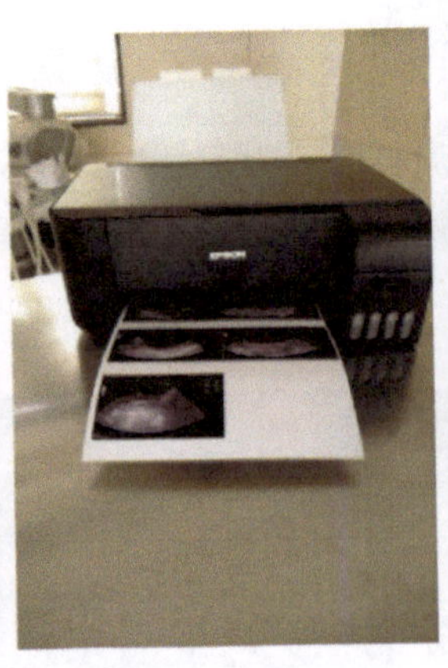

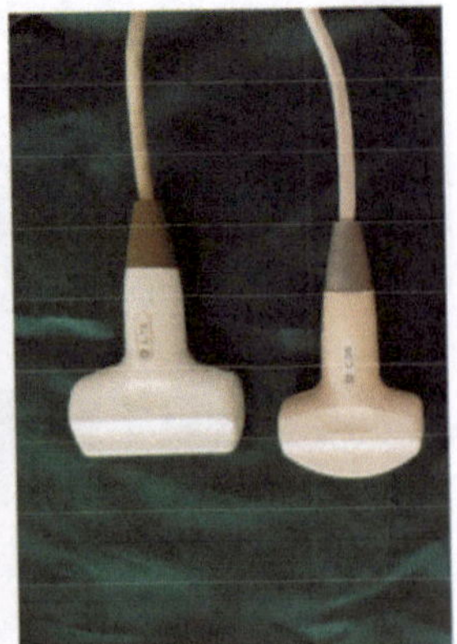

A B C

Figure 47: Ultrasound Machine (A), Printer (B) and (Probes (C).

During ultrasonography four types of error (errors due to perception, errors due to cognition, equipment related errors, inevitable errors or multifactorial errors) may creep in. The operator (person doing ultrasonographic examination) should be adequately trained and knowledgeable expert.

Hepatobilliary system

The echo texture of normal liver (without any pathology) is a mixed echo texture as shown in the Figure 48. Gall bladder (Figure 49) appears as a small fluid filled structure. The hepatic echo texture shows variations in different diseases of the liver. In acute disease, echotexture of the liver becomes more hypoechoic and in chronic disease, it becomes more hyperechoic. .Hepatic ultrasonography plays an important role in the diagnosis of acute (hepatitis/ hepatosis) and chronic liver diseases (hepatic insufficiency, fatty liver, cirrhosis, focal parenchymal lesions, masses, fluid filled cysts, abscess,) and biliary diseases (cholecystitis, mucocele, choleliths, biliary duct obstruction). In human medicine hepatic sonography is also used to evaluate portal venous phase to discriminate among benign and malignant nodules with a high sensitivity and specificity (Durot *et al.*, 2018). Portal hypertension or portal cava shunts can also be identified using Doppler evaluation of portal vein flow.

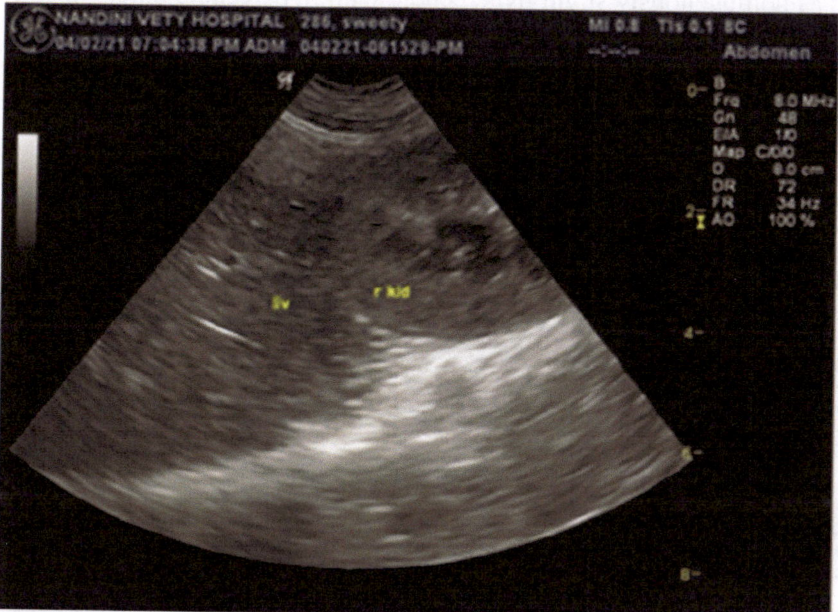

Figure 48: Sonogram of the normal liver of a healthy dog. Sonographically normal liver shows coarse echo texture (Courtesy Varshney, J.P.and Chaudhury, P.S. 2022).

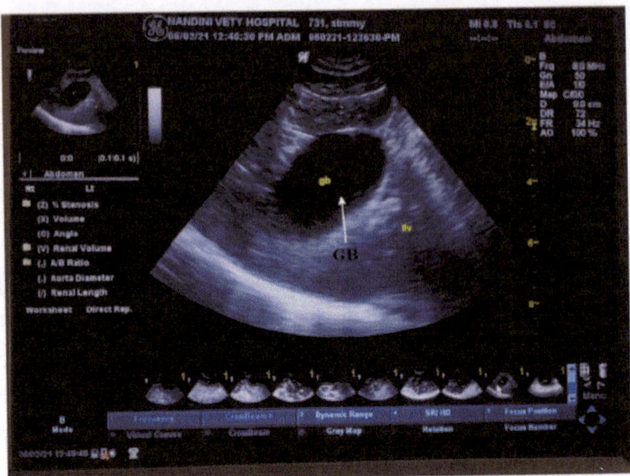

Figure 49: Sonogram of a dog showing gall bladder as a fluid filled organ marked with white arrow (Courtesy Varshney, J.P.and Chaudhury, P.S. 2022)

The Spleen

The spleen is always included in abdominal ultrasonography. Ultrasonogram of a spleen of a healthy dog is shown in the Figure 50. Sonographically the spleen appears as homogenously slight hyperechoic with hyperechoic outer capsule. The spleen is slightly more hyperechoic than the liver. Splenic ultrasound is indicated in cases of primary torsion, gastric volvulus where spleen may be involved in torsion, splenic masses and splenic rupture causing life threatening hemorrhages.

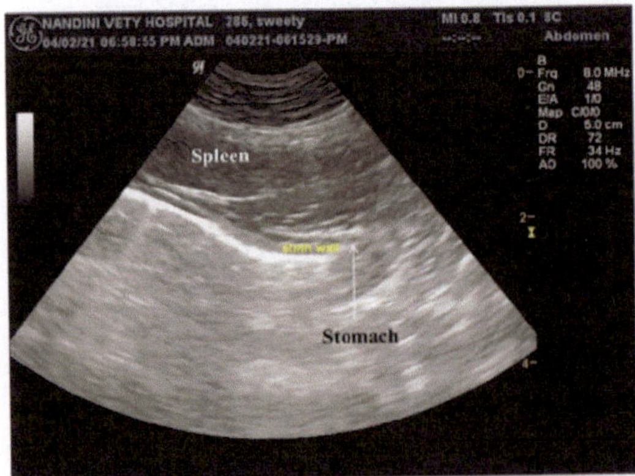

Figure 50: Sonogram of normal spleen of a dog. It is sonographically homogenously slight hyperechoic echotexture with hyperechoic outer capsule. The spleen is slightly hyperechoic than the liver (Courtesy Varshney, J.P.and Chaudhury ,P.S. 2022).

The Gastro-intestinal Tract

The gastro-intestinal sonography is performed to examine, stomach, small intestines and large intestines. Peristaltic movement can also be noted. The wall of the stomach and intestines (Figure 51) is made of five layers of alternating hyperechoic and hypoechoic echoes. From inner side to outer side, the gastric wall layers are: hyperechoic mucosal surface, hypoechoic mucosa, hyperechoic submucosa, hypoechoic muscularis propria and hyperechoic serosa. The Gastro-intestinal tract is sonographically evaluated for changes in wall thickness, intraluminal mass, length of lesion, integrity of the wall layers , bowel contents (fluid, gas, mucus alone or in combination), regional lymph nodes and peristalsis. While examining gastro-intestinal tract pancreatic area (pancreas, pancreatic duct, common bile duct and gall bladder) is also evaluated. Normal pancreas is sonographically not identifiable. However, diseased pancreas is sonographically visualized.

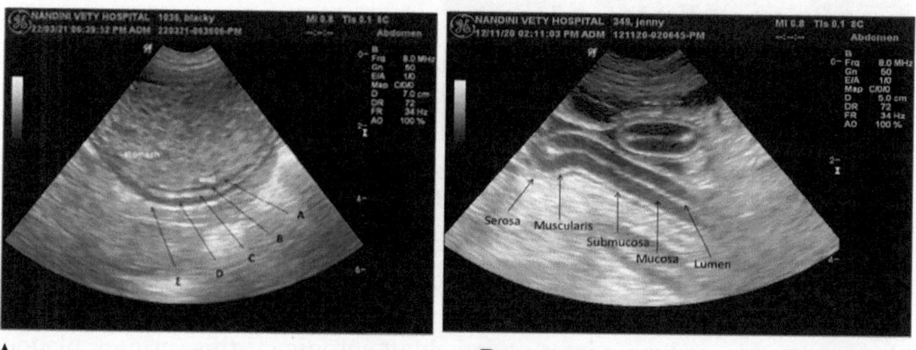

A B

Figure 51: Sonogram of the gastric wall **(A)** and intestinal wall **(B)** of healthy dogs. From inner side to outer side, the gastric wall layers (A) are: hyperechoic mucosal surface , hypoechoic mucosa, hyperechoic submucosa , hypoechoic muscularis propria , and hyperechoic serosa. The wall of the intestines also has five layers .From outside to inside , the intestinal wall layers are thin hyperechoic serosa, thin hypoechoic muscularis, thin hyperechoic submucosa, thickiest hypoechoic mucosa, and hyperechoic layer in the centre mucosal surface or lumen interface (Courtesy Varshney, J.P.and Chaudhury, P.S. 2022).

The Urinary System

Kidneys and urinary bladder are commonly subjected to sonography. Sonogram of a healthy kidney is shown in the Figure52. Kidneys are evaluated for its profile, pelvis dimension, alteration in vascularization, modification of cortical echogenicity, localized or diffused lesions and presence or absence of calculi. It also plays an important role in monitoring the progress in cases of chronic kidney disease. The technique is of diagnostic value in detecting primary or multiple nodular masses, cystic formation and its location, calculi and its location. Urethral lesions (obstruction) can also be identified.

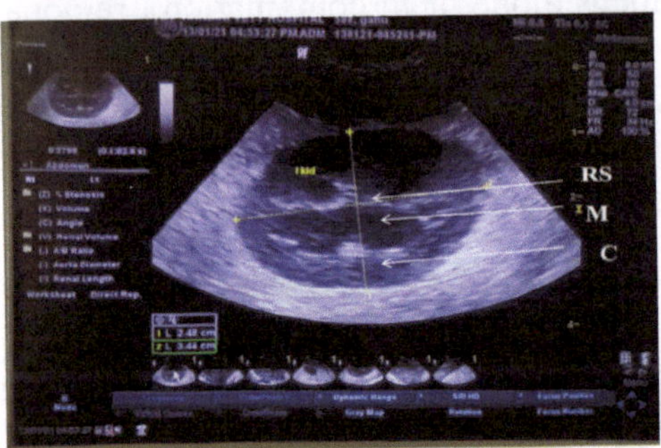

Figure 52: Sonogram of a normal kidney of an adult healthy dog showing renal pelvis, cortex and medulla. Renal cortex © is hyperechoic and renal medulla (M) is least echogenic. Renal sinus (RS)is more echogenic (Courtesy Varshney, J.P. and Chaudhary, P.S. 2022).

Sonographically the urinary bladder looks like a sac containing anechoic fluid and a hyperechoic bladder wall (Figure53). Sonography of the urinary bladder provides valuable information about chronic cystitis (urinary bladder wall of > 3 mm thickness), tumor, crystalluria (Figure54) , calculi and blood clot (haemorrhages in urinary bladder). Prostatic diseases such as benign hyperplasia of prostate, tumor, abscesses can also be identified in male dogs

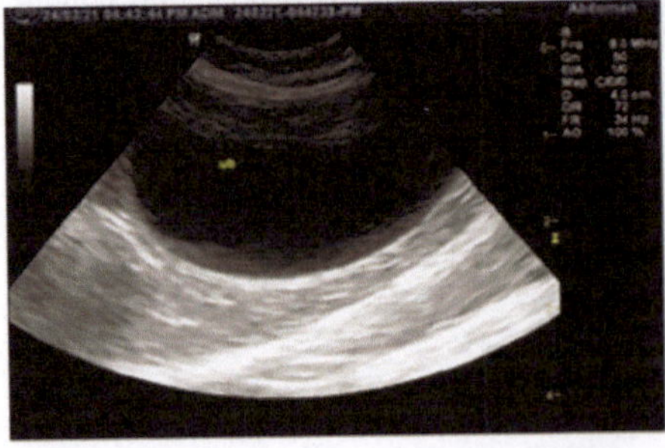

Figure 53: Sonogram of a healthy dog showing urinary bladder. Sonographically the urinary bladder looks like a sac containing anechoic fluid and a hyperechoic bladder wall (Courtesy Varshney, J.P. and Chaudhary, P.S. 2022).

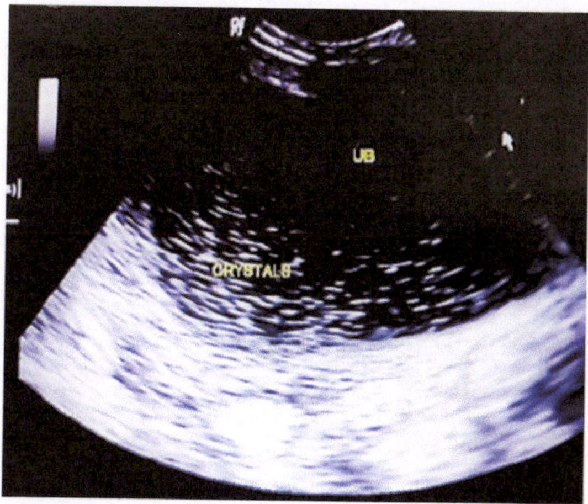

Figure 54: Sonogram of a dog showing crytalluria. Sonographically the crystals look like a hyper echoic particles of variable size sedimenting in the dependnt part of the bladder with distal acoustic shadowing .

The Adrenals

Adrenals are very small glandular structure. Left adrenal is peanut shaped while right adrenal is oval. Imaging of right adrenal is a challenging task because of its location (cranially adjacent to caudal vena cava) and air /food/ fluid filled gastrointestinal tract. Change in size, shape and echotexture of the adrenals in seen in pathological state.

Lymph Nodes

Lymph nodes in different anatomical locations are sonographically evaluated for their shape, echogenicity and vascularity for diagnosing inflammatory condition or malignancy.

Reproductive Tract

Ultrasonography of the reproductive tract of canines has become a routine practice to diagnose pregnancy (Figure55), to confirm foetal wellbeing, to confirm live/dead status of the foetus, to know ovarian status/phase, and to diagnose reproductive ailments (uterine, ovarian,) in females; and to diagnose diseases of prostate gland, cryptorchid, and testicular diseases in males. Non-gravid uterus is difficult to visualize in healthy bitches.

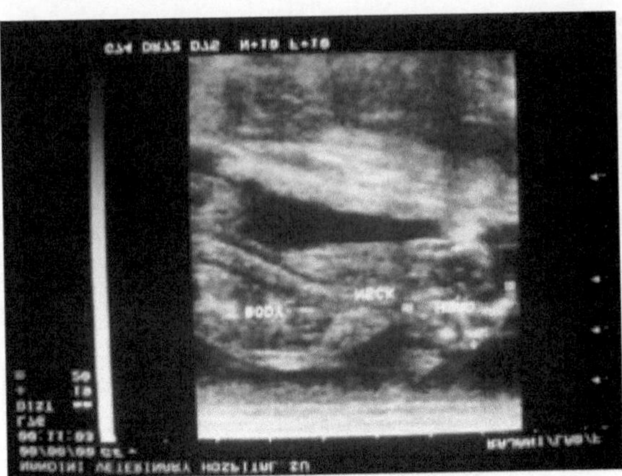

Figure 55: Sonogram of a bitch showing well developed fetus confirming pregnancy (*Courtesy* Varshney, J.P. and Chaudhary, P.S. 2022).

The Thorax

Beside heart, ultrasound of the thorax facilitates the imaging of lungs, pleura, mediastinum, chest wall and diaphragm .It can assist in the diagnosis of underlying causes of respiratory distress/dyspnea specially when thoracic radiograph is uncommitted . Identification of pulmonary and pleural diseases is also made easy by ultrasonographic examination. Thoracic ultrasound has limitations because of nearly total reflection of sound waves at gas interfaces. Further, deep pulmonary and mediastinal lesions poses difficulty in imaging. Visualization of peripheral pulmonary lesions and pleural fluid poses no difficulty. Lung ultrasound is becoming an effective tool in diagnosing left sided congestive heart failure in humans, dogs and cats and differentiating pulmonary edema of cardiac and non-cardiac origin. Thoracocentesis, aspiration of lung mass or consolidated lungs is facilitated with the application of thoracic ultrasound. Distinguishing fluid and soft tissues is also feasible with thoracic ultrasonography.

Musculoskeletal

Musculoskeletal sonography is a growing field in canine medicine because of increasing number of cases of soft tissue injuries. Cases of soft tissue injuries are increasing in dogs because of sports activities. The indications for musculoskeletal ultrasonography are injuries due to bicipital muscle tendon (tendinitis/partial rupture), avulsion of the distal bony insertion of the tendon, chronic myositis of ileopsoas muscles, muscles rupture, muscle neoformations (granuloma/abscess/neoplasia), osteoarthritis, and tendon/ligament diseases (inflammation, partial/complete rupture).

Thyroid and Parathyroid

Ultrasonographic imaging of thyroid and parathyroid is indicated in suspected cases of hyperthyroidism and hyperparathyroidism in dogs. It is also used to differentiate cases of primary hypothyroidism and euthyroidism. Thyroid gland has two lobes located on either side of the trachea on the ventral side of the neck. Parathyroids are very small glands located on crano-dorsal edge or caudal aspect of thyroid.

Echocardiography

Echocardiography (Figure 56) is the gold standard for assessing structure and function of the heart. It is cardiac ultrasonography. It is becoming an indispensible diagnostic technique for diagnosing congenital heart diseases, shunts, complex malformations, valvular heart diseases, cardiomyopathies, endocarditis, pericardial effusion, cor pulmonale and cardiac tumor. The diagnosis of these diseases was otherwise difficult before the advent of echocardiography. M -mode and color Doppler imaging is further improving our diagnostic skill. Evaluation of the heart involves real time B-mode, M-mode and Doppler echocardiography for better results.

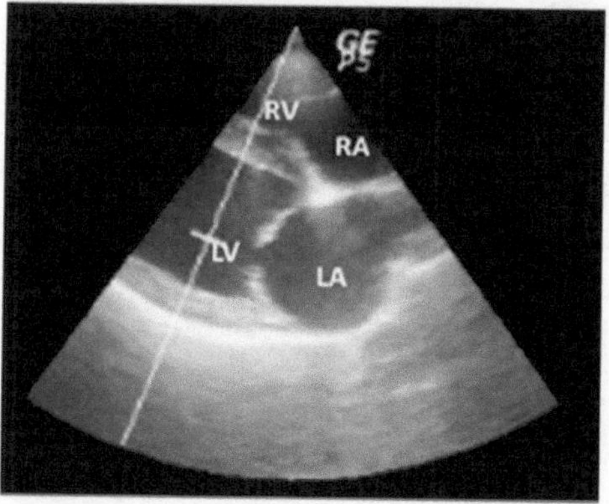

Figure 56: Echocardiogram of a healthy dog (right parasternal long axis view). Both atrium and ventricles can be seen. Left atrium,, right atrium, left ventricle and right ventricles are marked as LA, RA, LV and RV respectively (*Courtesy* Saini Neetu and Varshney, J.P.2022)

Endoscopy

It is an invasive technique to examine interior of body cavity or a hollow organ. The advent of fiber optic endoscope has made this technique a valuable tool in companion animal practice. The endoscopy is used to examine respiratory system (Bronchoscopy), esophagus (Esophagoscopy), stomach (Gastroscopy), small intestines (Enteroscopy), large intestines (Colonoscopy), peritoneal cavity (Laparoscopy), liver (laparoscopy), spleen (laparoscopy), pancreas (laparoscopy), urinary bladder (Cystoscopy) and joints (arthroscopy). The technique is also valuable in the removal of foreign bodies, taking biopsy, and for tumor therapy, Recently ultrathin endoscopes (2-3 mm diameter) have been developed for examining blood vessels. Endoscopes are of two types viz. rigid (laparoscope –Figure 57B, arthroscope) and flexible (gastroscope – Figure 57A, bronchoscope- Figure 57C). Rigid endoscope is used to examine abdominal cavity (laparoscope- Figure57). Flexible endoscopes are used to examine upper digestive tract such as esophagus and stomach, colon etc.

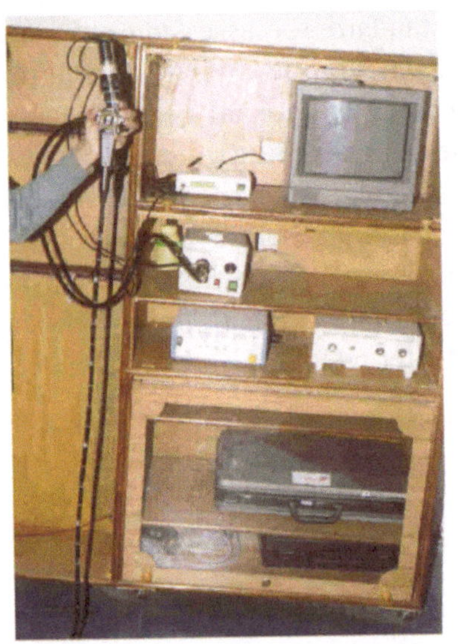

A

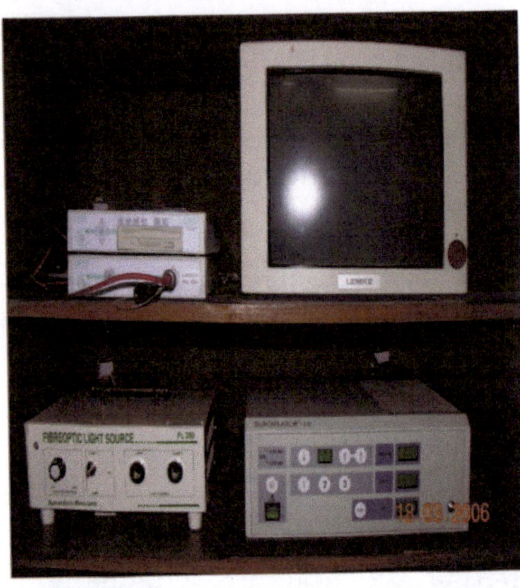

B

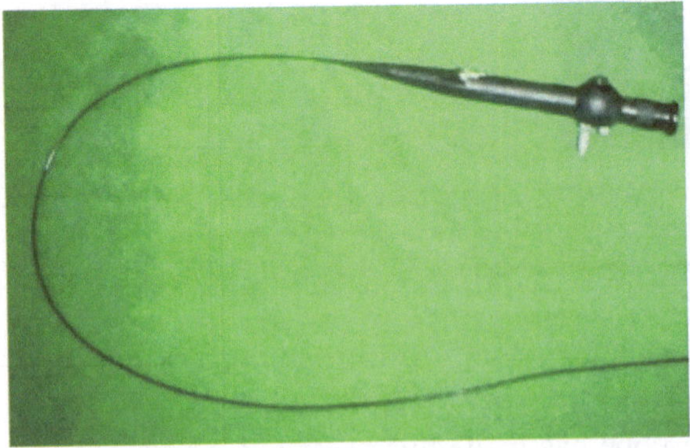

C

Figure 57: Showing different types of endoscopes. **A.** Gastroscope. **B.** Laparoscope. **C.** Bronchoscope.

Scintigraphy or Nuclear Medicine

Scintigraphy in veterinary medicine dates back to 1970's. Its principal use is in orthopedic conditions. Bone defects can be identified well before radiological detection. Its other uses are evaluation of vascular perfusion, pulmonary ventilation, cardiac output damage and to detect intrathoracic pathology.

References

Durot, I., Wilson, S.R., and Willmann, J.K.(2018). Contrast-enhanced ultrasound of malignant liver lesions. Abdom. Radiol. 43:819–847.

Saini Neetu and Varshney,J.P. (2022). Cardiac Ultrasound. In: Ultrasound in Veterinary Medicine. Fundamentals and Application.NIPA Genx Electronic Resources and Solutions P.Ltd. New Delhi-110034

Varshney, J.P. and Chaudhary, P.S. (2022). Ultrasound of the Liver and Gall bladder. In: Ultrasound in Veterinary Medicine. Fundamentals and Application.NIPA Genx Electronic Resources and Solutions P.Ltd. New Delhi-110034

Varshney, J.P. and Chaudhary, P.S. (2022). Ultrasound of the Spleen . In: Ultrasound in Veterinary Medicine. Fundamentals and Application.NIPA Genx Electronic Resources and Solutions P.Ltd. New Delhi-110034 .

Varshney,J.P. and Chaudhary, P.S. (2022). Ultrasound of the Stomach . In: Ultrasound in Veterinary Medicine. Fundamentals and Application.NIPA Genx Electronic Resources and Solutions P.Ltd. New Delhi-110034 .

Varshney, J.P. and Chaudhary, P.S. (2022). Ultrasound of the Intestines. In: Ultrasound in Veterinary Medicine. Fundamentals and Application.NIPA Genx Electronic Resources and Solutions P.Ltd. New Delhi-110034

Varshney, J.P. and Chaudhary, P.S. (2022). Ultrasound of the Urinary Tract. In: Ultrasound in Veterinary Medicine. Fundamentals and Application.NIPA Genx Electronic Resources and Solutions P.Ltd. New Delhi-110034 .

Varshney, J.P. and Chaudhary, P.S. (2022). Ultrasound of the Reproductive Tract. In: Ultrasound in Veterinary Medicine. Fundamentals and Application.NIPA Genx Electronic Resources and Solutions P.Ltd. New Delhi-110034.

7

Clinical Diagnostic Techniques in Cardiology

Last few decades have witnessed an increasing number of pets attending clinics/hospitals for cardiac care because of changed life style of owners as well as pets, more awareness of the owners and an increase in number of veterinary medical specialist with better diagnostic facilities. Cardiac failure and cardiac arrest are the two important outcome of cardiac diseases with variable treatment result. Heart functioning is affected not only in primary diseases of heart but also in diseases of organs other than the heart. Without correct diagnosis of cardiac abnormalities, treatment may be futile with a fatal outcome. Nowadays diagnosis of cardiac abnormalities is facilitated with the aid of modern diagnostic technology. Though, clinical examination plays a significant role in the diagnosis of cardiac diseases, yet clinical significance of murmurs and /or arrhythmias is baffling without further investigations. Sometimes non-cardiac ailments also manifest symptoms mimicking heart diseases. As cough, tiredness, weakness, dyspnea, respiratory crackling are also evident in lung diseases and need differentiation whether these signs are due to cardiac or pulmonary origin. Before the advent of electrocardiography much reliance was paid to ancillary approach (analyzing history, clinical symptoms and clinical examination) that lacks differentiating ability of various cardiac diseases. Nowadays it is possible to evaluate animals at risk of cardiac diseases even when clinical manifestations are not apparent. Recent advances in cardiology during last few decades, most notably in the areas of diagnostic imaging and biomarkers have considerably improved our diagnostic skill in differentiating various heart diseases of which diagnosis was unimaginable during early 20th century. History, detail clinical examination, chest radiography, vertebral heart score, electrocardiography, continuous Holter monitoring, echocardiography, Doppler echocardiography, trans-esophageal echocardiography, angiocardiography, cardiac catheterization, pulmonary capillary wedge pressure measurement, central venous pressure measurement, endomyocardial biopsy, nuclear cardiology, pneumopericardiography, oxymetry, and monitoring of cardiac biomarkers play pivotal role in the diagnosis of cardiac ailments. All diagnostic techniques have their own limitations. No single diagnostic approach is self-sufficient to achieve the diagnostic goal. Hanky-panky and casual approach is unrewarding. In fact a systematic approach is required to ascertain the diagnosis of heart diseases. A bird eye view of different diagnostic techniques, in vogue, for evaluating heart is presented below for sensitizing and making the students and general practitioners familiar with diagnostic approaches in cardiac cases so that cardiac patients are timely refereed to subject matter specialist.

History and Clinical Examination

Despite technical ability of modern diagnostic tools, obtaining and examining history in detail and conducting physical examination is the most important and desirable first step in the direction of making a correct diagnosis of cardiac ailments. These basic examinations provide important leads and direction to undertake further specific examinations for making exact and correct diagnosis. History of nocturnal coughing in dogs arises suspicion of cardiac involvement but it does not always reflect heart disease. Neither all dogs with heart failure cough nor all coughing dogs have cardiac disease. Coughing episodes worsening with exercise/ excitement/ or at night in a lying animal creates strong suspicion of cardiac cough. Exercise intolerance, cyanosis, sudden fainting, marked weakness, inappetance and weight loss are the other historical narration by the owners. These are related to reduce cardiac output and cannot be taken for granted for heart ailment only. History of abdominal distension has also been speculated for cardiac disease but it is also a reflection of hepatomegaly, splenomegaly, and renal failure as well as of right heart failure. Amongst heart diseases, large and giant breeds are more susceptible to cardiomyopathies while small and toy breeds are more susceptible to valvular heart problems.

As other organ dysfunctions are manifested with signs and symptoms, cardiac ailments are also manifested with many symptoms. The clinical symptoms in dogs with heart diseases are mainly due to forward failure, backward failure and arrhythmias. Early clinical signs of heart failure are vague and nonspecific mainly because of decreased cardiac output. As heart failure progresses, clinical signs start appearing. Mucus membrane color changes due to forward and/or backward failure. Reduced cardiac output leads to lower rectal temperature and cold extremities. Capillary refill time increases. Jugular vein distension and positive hepato-jugular reflex may be detected. Coughing, dyspnea, wheezes and crackling may be evident due to pulmonary edema. Decreased appetite may lead to cardiac cachexia. Femoral arterial pulse becomes weak with pulse deficit. Abdominal distension and hind limb edema may become appreciable. In advance stage, arrhythmias, murmurs and muffling heart sound are also detected. To appreciate and detect these changes a thorough physical examination is very vital. The physical examination involves inspection (looking for abducted elbow, jugular distension or pulse, edema of ventral abdomen or limbs, tachypnea /dyspnea), vital indices (changes in rectal temperature, pulse, respiration, mucus membrane color, capillary refill time), palpation (ascertain position of apex beat, presence or absence of precordial thrill, femoral pulse, ascites, hepatomegaly) and auscultation (to detect changes in heart rate and rhythm, intensity of heart sounds, murmurs or abnormal respiratory sounds). Heart is to be auscultated at all valve areas (details given in Chapter 1). Heart sounds are more intense in young dogs, thin dogs, and dogs suffering from fever, hyperthyroidism or anemia. While its intensity decreases in obese dogs, dogs with pleural or pericardial effusions. Auscultation of the heart is also necessary to detect arrhythmias and murmurs. Pathological murmurs are detected in cases of valvular insufficiency, valvular stenosis, interatrial or interventricular septal defects, patent ductus arteriosus (PDA) or defect of great vessels. Murmurs are graded as grade 1 to grade 6 on the basis of their intensity and location. Grade 1 murmurs are localized, very soft and detected on prolonged auscultation. Grade 2 murmurs are almost similar to grade 1 but are detected easily. Grade 3 murmurs are moderately intense and detected at more than one place. Grade 4 murmurs are similar to grade 3 murmurs but are detected at many places in both side chest (left and right). Loud murmurs heard over point of maximum intensity with precordial thrill are graded as grade 5 murmur. Grade 6 murmurs are very loud and are associated with precordial thrill

Blood Pressure Monitoring

Blood pressure is the measure of force that heart uses to pump the blood in arteries around body. There is two type of blood pressure viz systolic (when blood is pumped in arteries during cardiac systole) and diastolic (when the heart is in diastole and receiving the blood). For non-invasive measurement of blood pressure in clinical practice in canines, Doppler ultrasonic flow detector, oscillometry technique and auscultative technique are being used. The major limitation of non-invasive measurement of blood pressure in canines is its inaccuracy particularly in hypotensive patients. Blood pressure monitoring is indicated in dogs with heart disease, renal disease, endocrinopathies, and syncope and in dehydration. Blood pressure monitoring is valuable indicator of ventricular wall stress and myocardial oxygen consumption.

Auscultative Method

In auscultative method, the dog is restrained in right lateral recumbency and Velcro cuff is applied over hind limb on cranial tibial artery at the distal medial aspect of tibia (Figure58). The width of the cuff should be around 30-40 % of the circumference of the fore limb, hind limb or tail from which arterial blood pressure is being measured. The cuff is inflated with air using hand bulb (as shown in the Figure 58). The pressure varies in the cuff. The systolic and diastolic arterial pressures are indicated by the appearance of palpable beat with cuff deflation or appearance of throbbing of manometer or sound and ceasing of throbbing or sound respectively.

Oscillometric Method

Devices measuring blood pressure based on oscillometric method are automated providing estimates of heart rate; and systolic, mean, and diastolic arterial blood pressure. These devices inflate the cuff automatically until arterial blood flow is impeded. As deflation of cuff begins slowly, the oscillometer measures the mean arterial blood pressure as the value at which the pressure oscillations in the cuff have maximum amplitude and an algorithm is used to compute systolic and diastolic arterial BP values from the measured mean arterial blood pressure (Williamson and Leone, 2012).

Doppler Ultrasonic Flow Detector

This method (Figure 59) of measuring blood pressure is based on the similar principle of auscultatory method except that it uses a distally placed flow detector rather than stethoscope. Ultrasonic gel is liberally applied on the surface of the Doppler probe and then it is placed over a peripheral artery (hairs of the area should be clipped). An occlusive cuff is placed proximally and a sphygmomanometer is used to inflate the cuff until blood flow, and therefore systolic arterial BP, is impeded, causing the audible signal to disappear (Clarke *et al*., 2014). The cuff is slowly deflated and the cuff pressure at which the first audible sound returns suggests the value of systolic arterial blood pressure. The technique is minimally invasive, cheap, and easy to use.

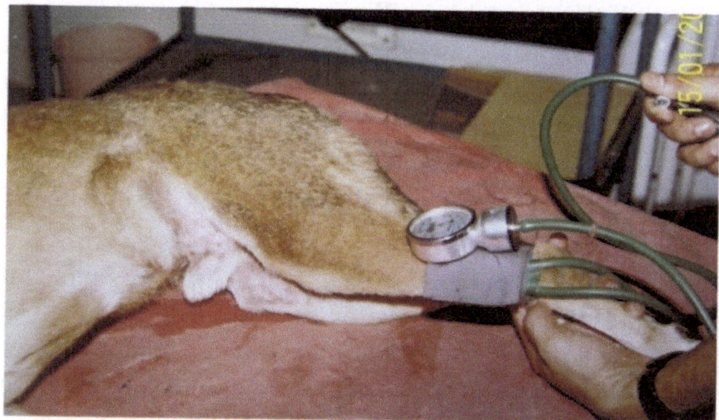

Figure 58: Blood pressure measurement by indirect technique using a small Velcro cuff (5 x 22 cm size) tied over left hind leg on cranial tibial artery at distal medial aspect of tibia and aneroid sphygmomanometer. The hand bulb coupled to aneroid pressure gauge calibrated in mm of mercury (Hg) is used to inflate and vary the pressure in the cuff. The systolic and diastolic arterial pressures are indicated by the appearance of palpable beat with cuff deflation or appearance of throbbing of manometer or sound and ceasing of throbbing or sound respectiuvely (Courtesy Varshney, J.P.2020)

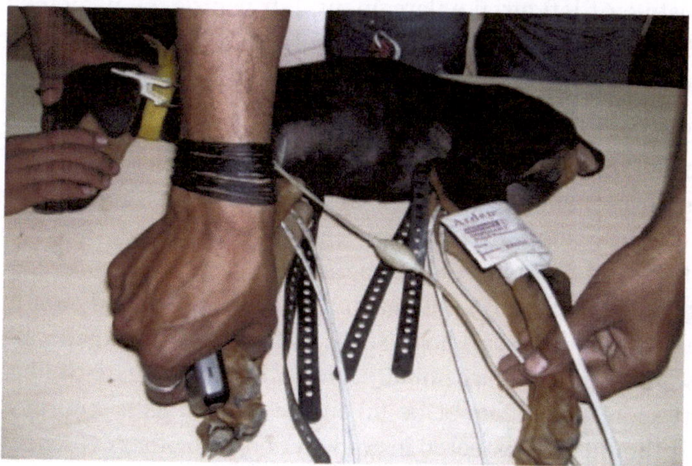

Figure 59: Blood pressure measurement by indirect technique using Ultrasonic Doppler Sensing device. (*Courtesy* Varshney, J.P.2020).

Thoracic Radiography

Thoracic radiography is of diagnostic value in dogs with congestive heart failure. Chamber enlargements can also be detected in radiographs. In all suspected cases of heart failure at least two views (right lateral and ventro dorsal) should be taken for assessment. Thoracic radiographs should be taken with high kilovoltage peak (kvp) and low milliamperes (mAs) at the peak of inspiration. In healthy dogs, ventricles occupy three intercostal space. Heart extends from 3rd to 6th intercostal space touching nearly diaphragm caudally. In heart radiographic silhouette, right atrium and right ventricle makes the cranial border; and left atrium and left ventricle make the caudal border. Both atria, pulmonary artery, aorta and cranial and caudal vena cava are on the dorsal side of the heart.

Right lateral radiographs revealing pulmonary edema (fluid opacity) in dorso-caudal hilar region (Figure 45) are suggestive of congestive heart failure in most of the cases. The edema is fluid accumulation in the interstitium and /or the pulmonary alveoli. When edema is detected in dosrso caudal hilar region of the lungs, congestive heart failure is almost certain. Thoracic radiographs can also suggest chamber enlargement, great vessel enlargement, heartworm disease, and pericardial or pleural effusions. In ventro-dorsal radiographs reduction in right heart to right chest wall distance and reduction in left heart to left chest wall distance is suggestive of right ventricular enlargement and left ventricular enlargement respectively. Bulges at 2 to 3 o'clock position , 3 to 5 o'clock position (with rounding) and 9-11 o'clock position of cardiac silhouette are suggestive of left atrial enlargement, left ventricle enlargement and right atrium enlargement respectively. A reverse D configuration of cardiac silhouette is suggestive of right ventricle enlargement.

Vertebral heart score (VHS), calculated on the lateral thoracic radiographs (Figure 60), also provides information about cardiac size. Long axis (from the carina of the main bronchus to the apex of the heart) and short axis of cardiac silhouette (at the widest part of the heart) are measured. The axis measurements are then transferred to the vertebrae starting from cranial edge of T4 .The number of vertebrae fall under each axis are counted and sum up to find vertebral heart score. Vertebral heart score exceeding 10.5 is generally is generally suggestive of heart enlargement. Being a rough estimate of heart size, vertebral heart score alone cannot be taken for granted as a criteria of heart enlargement. It should be considered in conjunction with other evidences.

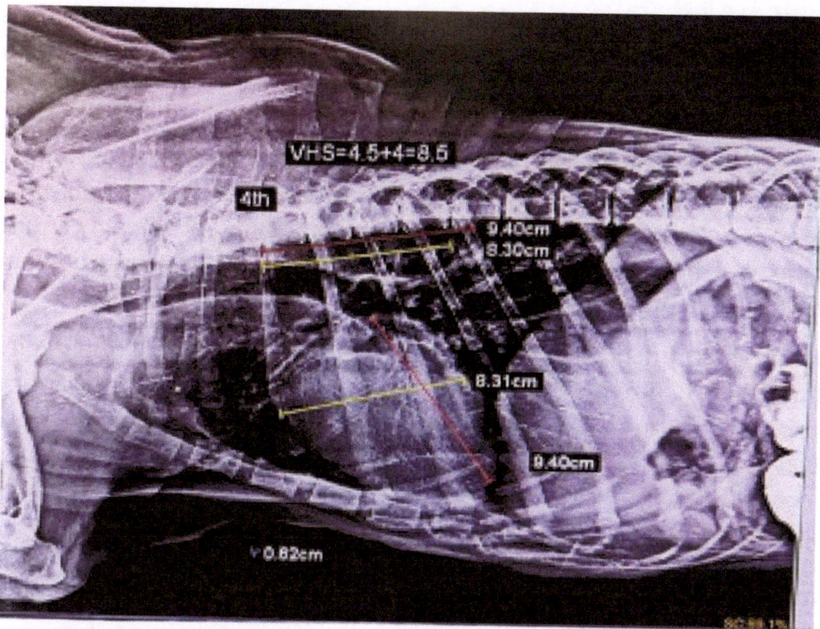

Figure 60: Right lateral radiograph of a dog showing measurements for vertebral heart score. Red line denotes long axis and yellow line denotes short axis of the cardiac silhouette. These measurements are then transferred to the vertebrae starting from cranial edge of T4 vertebra and then the number of vertebrae fall under each axis are counted and sum up to find vertebral heart score. In the above case VHS is 8.5.

Electrocardiography

Electrocardiography, non-invasive diagnostic technique, is routinely employed for cardiac evaluation both in human and canine medicine. Neither all changes in electrocardiogram are suggestive of cardiac pathology nor does a normal electrocardiogram rule out cardiac abnormalities. Electrocardiography is an essential technique for the diagnosis of arrhythmias (disturbances of heart rate and/or rhythm). In canines, an abnormal electrocardiogram may also suggest the side of the heart affected. This diagnostic technique is of great value in evaluating the heart in health and diseases. Nevertheless, it cannot be taken as a last tool in itself for the diagnosis of cardiac diseases. It may provide lead for further investigations. The technique has its own limitations in the diagnosis of heart diseases as it cannot detect mechanical status of the heart; diseases of cardiac valves, coronary arteries, endocardium and pericardium. An electrocardiogram (ECG) should always be interpreted as a part of clinical findings in conjunction with history, and the results of other cardiac evaluation techniques. Details of the technique are given in chapter 5.

Electrocardiographic evaluation of the heart should always be considered as a part of examination in cases with arrhythmias (tachycardia, bradycardia or irregular heartbeat, missing beats), shock, syncope, sudden dyspnea, seizures, cardiac murmurs, increased area of heart auscultation, renal disease, endocrinopathies (Addition's disease, Cushing's syndrome, thyroid dysfunctions), systemic diseases (pyometra, pancreatitis, uremia, neoplasms), acid-base and/ or ionic imbalances. The fact that sometimes significant cardiac disease may not be associated with definite changes in electrocardiogram should always be kept in mind.

For detecting intermittent arrhythmias, a 24 hour Holter electrocardiography is recommended. It provides a continuous 24 hours monitoring of cardiac electrical activity during normal daily activities, strenuous exercise or sleep. Holter electrocardiography is desirable and valuable technique in dogs with syncope wherein routine resting electrocardiogram and laboratory investigations generally remain inconclusive.

Echo-cardiography

Echo-cardiography is also a non-invasive diagnostic technique being used for evaluating the heart (chamber dimensions, valve configuration, motion and functioning, wall thickness, wall motion, mass in the heart etc.) and its surrounding structures. This technique can take care of the lacunae with electrocardiography. It is indicated for the diagnosis of differentiating cardiomyopathies, valvular diseases, pericarditis, pericardial effusion, pleural effusion and vessel diseases. It is highly sophisticated and expert dependent technique.

Cardiac Biomarkers

Cardiac biomarkers are comparatively a new step in diagnostic cardiology both in human and canine medicine and their use is increasing not only in clinical practice but also in research. These diagnostic methods are non-invasive and precise. The aim of cardiac markers is to detect myocardial damage, induced due to heart diseases, at the earliest. Biochemical markers now play an important role in the detection of cardiac disease, risk stratification and therapy monitoring. Although a number of biochemical markers (aspartate aminotransferase, lactic dehydrogenase and its isoenzyme –LD1, creatinine kinase and its isoenzyme MB, myoglobin, cardiac troponins –cTn-I, C-reactive protein, and cardiac natriuretic peptides-NT pro BNP) are being monitored to assess the myocardial damage in humans with heart diseases, only two biomarkers (cTn-I and NT pro BNP) have shown promise in diagnosing cardiac insult owing to cardiomyopathy or valvular heart diseases in canine cardiology. Cardiac Troponin-I (cTn-I) is a fundamental component of cardiomyocytes and is released in response to cardiac muscle insult (cardiac muscle remodeling or damage). Cardiac troponin- I is considered as a very sensitive biomarker of physical or metabolic myocardial injury, myocardial ischemia, or necrosis in humans with a cardiac specificity of 100%. Its level in serum increases in a biphasic manner after 4 to 6 hours of acute myocardial cell injury. Minor myocardial injury cannot be detected by electrocardiography (ECG) or echocardiography as their sensitivity is poor. An early diagnosis of myocardial injury is very important for an effective treatment and better prognosis. cTn-I is 100% specific for the heart. In healthy dogs its normal level is very low (0.03 to 0.07 ng/ml) or undetectable by current assay methods. At present both qualitative (Figure61) and quantitative estimation methods for cTn-I are available. An increase in the level of cTn-I is suggestive of myocardial injury but do not ascertain the cause and mechanism of cardiac insult. Troponin levels can rise with very small amounts of myocardial cell damage.

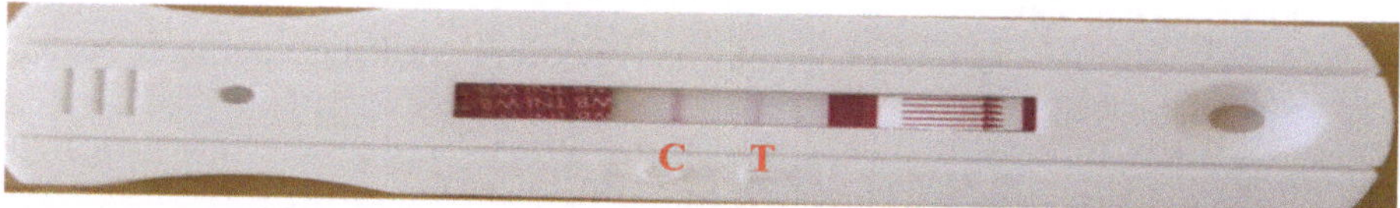

Figure 61: Cardiac Troponin-I test kit for the qualitative estimation of cTn-I level to detect cardiac insult. Appearance of purple colored line, in test region 'T' and pinkish purple line in the control region 'C' indicates that the sample is reactive to Troponin-I . Difference in the intensity of color between 'C' and 'T' is due to variations in Tn-I concentrations. The test can detect cTn-I in serum/plasma/whole blood as low as 0.3 ng/ml.

Cardiac troponin-I is usually released when the disease process is advanced. There is another cardiac biomarker BNP that is released in the early stage of cardiac insult. This biomarker was originally isolated from pig brain. NT pro-BNP is found in ventricle and is released in to circulation upon cardiac injury. It has potential to detect the dogs at the risk of heart disease or heart failure in the early stage. Healthy dogs have very low level (4.1386 to 16.5543 pmol/L) of NT-pro BNP and it seems to be a good indicator of differentiating severe respiratory distress of heart or lung origin.

Aspartate dehydrogenase (AST), creatine kinase (CK), lactate dehydrogenase (LDH) and myoglobin (M) are other biomarkers in use in cases of myocardial infarction and heart failure in humans. These biomarkers suffer from lack of specificity and damage is detected after establishment of the disease. Researches are continuing to develop better biomarkers that can detect the myocardial insult in the beginning of the myocardial stretch or damage or remodeling. Pro inflammatory-cytokines such as interleukin IL-1, IL-6, and TNF- α (Hedayat *et al.*, 2010), ST-2 (suppression of tumorigenicity 2), osteopontin and cardioprotrophin-1 (Jongasaki *et al.*,2000) and TNF- α (Schober, 2005), new generation biomarkers, are being investigated for detecting myocardial insult at the earliest for better management of heart failure. Though, these biomarkers have potential to detect cardiac insult, do not indicate the cause and type of cardiac muscle damage.

References

Clarke, K.W., Trim, C.M. and Hall, L.W. (2014). Patient monitoring and clinical measurement. In: Veterinary Anesthesia. Clarke, K.W., Trim, C.M. and Hall, L.W. (Eds.). 11th edn. St. Louis, Missouri: Elsevier pp. 30–38.

Hedayat, M., Mahmoudi, M.J., Rose, N.R. and Rezaei N (2010). Proinflammatory cytokines in heart failure: double edged swords. Heart Fail Rev 15:543–562.

Jongasaki ,M., Tachibana, I. and Luchner, A. (2000). Augmented cardiotrophin-I in experimental congestive heart failure. Circulation 101:14–17.

Schober (2005) Biochemical markers of cardiovascular disease. In: Textbook of VeterinaryMedicine. Ettimger, S.J. and Feldman, E.C. (eds.) vol 2. Elsevier, St. Louis, pp 940–948.

Varshney, J.P. (2020). Electrocardiography in Veterinary Medicine. Springer Nature, Singapore, Pte.Ltd.

Williamson, J.A. and Leone, S. (2012). Noninvasive arterial blood pressure monitoring. In: Advanced Monitoring and Procedures for Small Animal Emergency and Critical Care. Burkitt Creedon, J.M. and Davis, H. (Eds.). 1st edn. Wiley Blackwell Ames, Iowa. pp. 134–144.

8

Clinical Diagnostic Techniques in Dermatology

The prevalence of skin diseases in dogs is high throughout the world. Skin diseases are one of the main clinical complaint with which dogs and cats are presented at clinics. Skin diseases are numerous and have wide range of underlying etiology ranging from non-specific cause, infections (bacterial, viral, fungal. yeast), hormonal, nutritional to immunological causes. Most of the skin diseases are clinically manifested with focal or diffuse alopecia, itching, papules, pustules, erythema, scaling, scabs, lumps, unpleasant smell, rashes, urticarial plaques, dandruff, hot spots or excessive licking (Figure62) making the straight forward diagnosis a difficult task especially in dogs and cats with chronic dermatological disease. Therefore, detail examination of history and clinical manifestations followed by a series of diagnostic test is mandatory to identify the underlying disease and to undertake rational treatment to avoid unnecessary use of drugs, to reduce the cost of treatment, to hasten recovery, to increase cure rate and to avoid owners' frustration. Although most of the tests being conducted in canine and feline dermatology appear simple, it still requires clinical and professional acumen; proper collection of the sample and its processing; and correct handling. The fact that no test is cent-percent reliable should always be kept in mind especially when the dog/cat is exhibiting obvious lesions but test result is negative. Flea combing or brushing, acetate tape, skin scrapping, impression smear, trichogram, cytology, Woods lamp, intradermal allergen test, and culture (bacterial and fungal) examination are the most common clinical diagnostic techniques being employed in canine and feline dermatology.

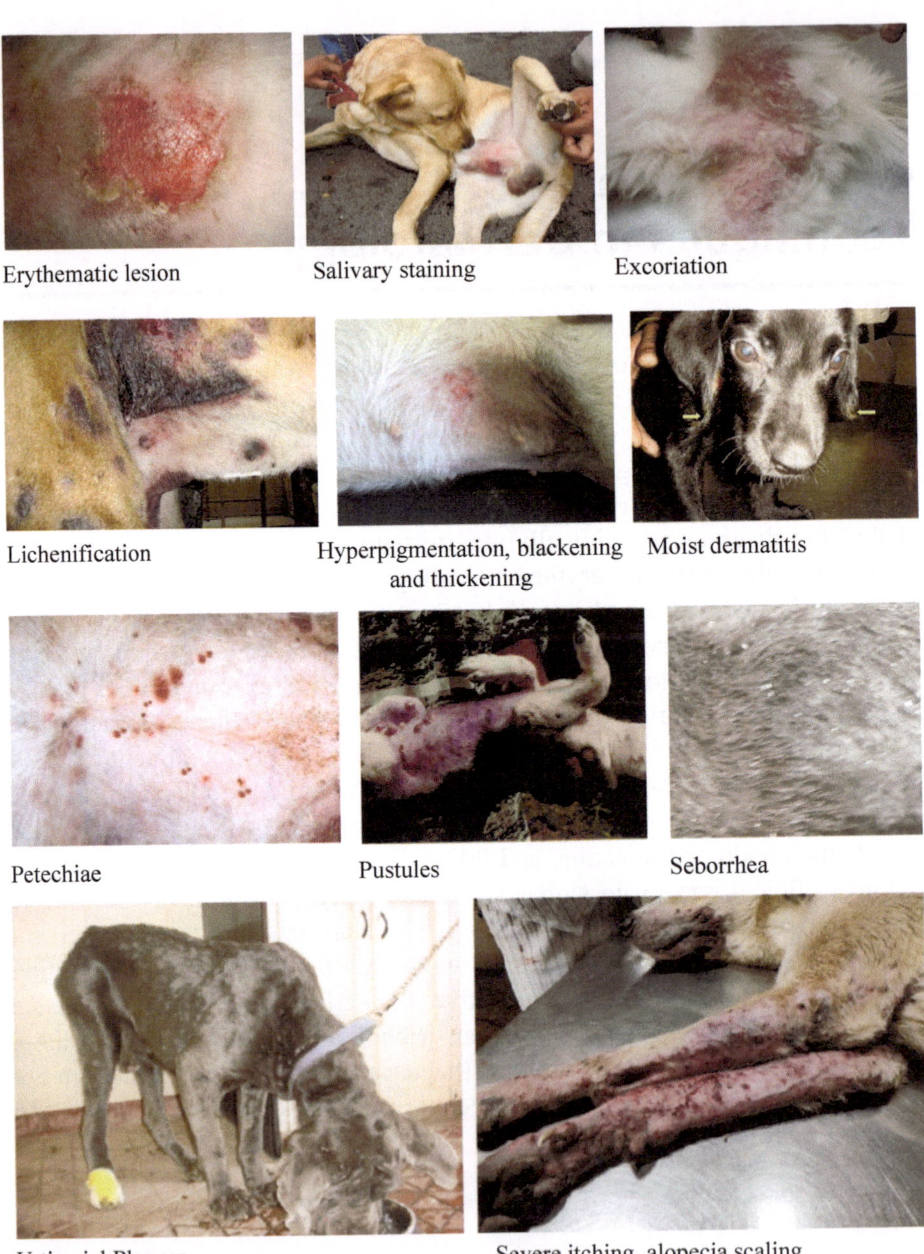

Erythematic lesion | Salivary staining | Excoriation

Lichenification | Hyperpigmentation, blackening and thickening | Moist dermatitis

Petechiae | Pustules | Seborrhea

Urticarial Plaques (Courtesy Varshney, J.P.2023) | Severe itching, alopecia,scaling and bleeding (self mutilation)

Figure 62: Showing different types of skin lesions.

Flea Combing/Coat Brushing Test

Flea infestation (Figure 63) is very common in dogs and cats and can be easily detected when adult fleas are present on the body. When fleas are in small number, the diagnosis of flea infestation with naked eyes becomes difficult. In that situation flea combing or coat brushing test is of great assistance. Flea combing or coat brushing test is very simple and underutilized dermatological technique. It has great screening potential for detecting flea feces or flea dirt, ectoparasites, eggs and follicular abnormalities. The test is conducted by combing or brushing the animal over the black or brown paper. The hairs from the collected material (hairs and debris) are separated and placed in petri dish for examination with Wood's lamp and a portion is mounted in liquid paraffin with a cover slip for examination under microscope. The technique is indicated in patients with intense itching, seborrhea or previous history of fleas' infestation. Lice, nits, *Cheyletiella* and fragmented flea feces can be identified that is otherwise missed macroscopically. Combs or brushes need to be properly washed after each use and be kept in a container having a disinfectant to avoid contamination and transmission of infectious agents.

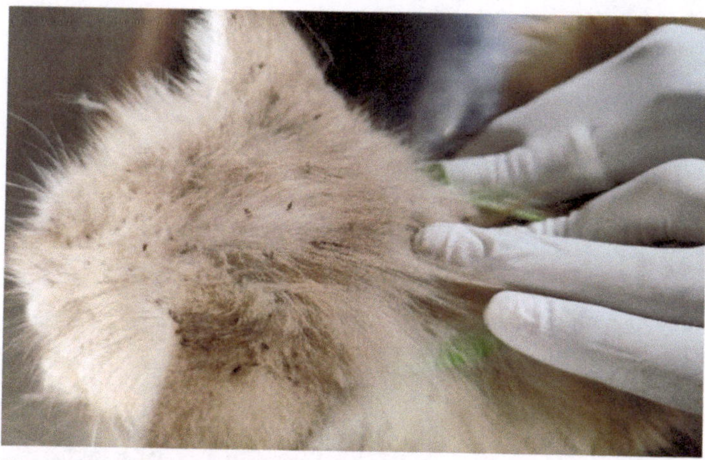

Figure 63: Showing Fleas Infestation.

Paper Towel Test

The test is conducted for looking flea dirt in material collected from brushing test. Many times fleas are not seen, but the presence of flea dirt (feces) indicates flea infestation. The flea dirt is composed of digested blood. When flea dirt is dissolved in water and put on white paper towel, it leaves behind red-brownish stain on the paper suggesting the possibility of flea infestation. This test provides the indirect evidence of flea infestation.

Skin Scrapping Test

Skin scrapping test is necessary in cases where mite infestation is suspected and less invasive test is negative. It is primarily indicated to detect surface (scabies) and burrowing (demodex) mites or other mite such as *Cheyletiella, Notoedres* and *Otodectes*. Skin scrappings (Figure 64) are collected using a blunt blade (no.10), dipped in mineral oil, in the direction of the hair growth. The first few scrapes are superficial then subsequent scrapes are deep. Deep skin scraping are required for detection of the demodex (Figure 65 A and B) as these mites live in the hair follicles. Squeezing the skin prior to scraping increases the chance of detecting the mites. For scabies (Figure 65 C and D), multiple scrapping, both superficial and deep, in non-excoriated areas are to be collected. The collected scraping are transferred on to a slide , mixed with a drop of liquid paraffin , covered with a cover slip and are examined under low power (10X). The liquid paraffin does not kill the mite and subtle movement may help to locate its position.

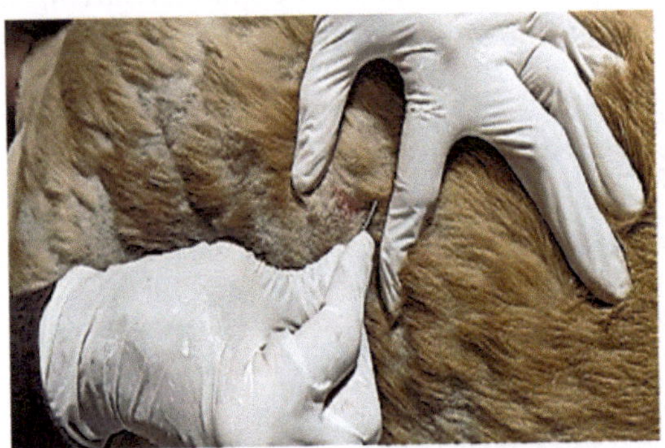

Figure 64: Showing skin scrapping test in a dog.

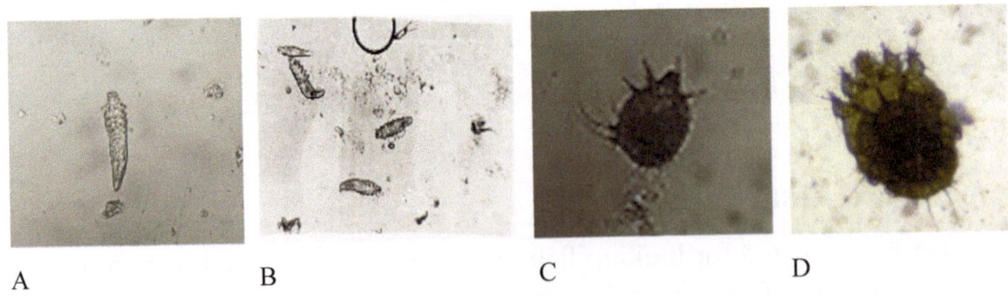

Figure65. Showing *Demodex canis* mite (A and B) and Sarcoptes mites (C and D)

Acetate Tape Strip Test

Acetate tape strip test (Figure 66 A) is a quick, informative, inexpensive and versatile test in dermatology. It is indicated in the diagnosis of superficial pyoderma, bacterial overgrowth, some parasitic and autoimmune diseases. It is most commonly employed in the diagnosis of dermatitis caused by Malassezia or bacterial overgrowth. Test is performed by repeatedly pressing several pieces (about 10 cm length) of acetate tape on to the surface of the affected skin, particularly of greasy areas, and then taking it out. Acetate tape can be stained as a glass slide, rinsed and pressed to a microscopic slide (Figure 66 B) with the sticky surface on the slide. Unstained tapes can also be examined in a similar manner as stained tapes.

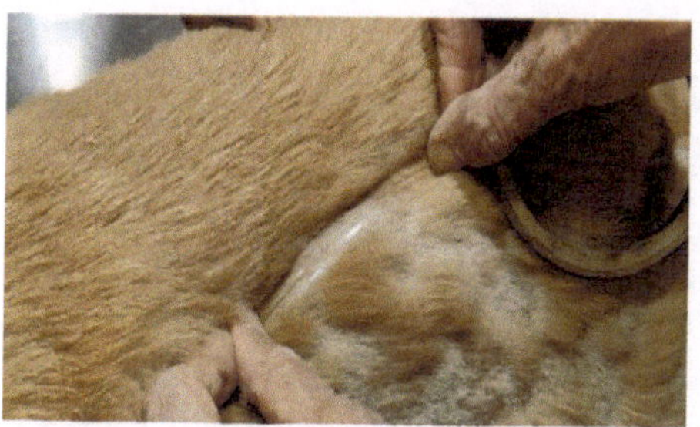

A

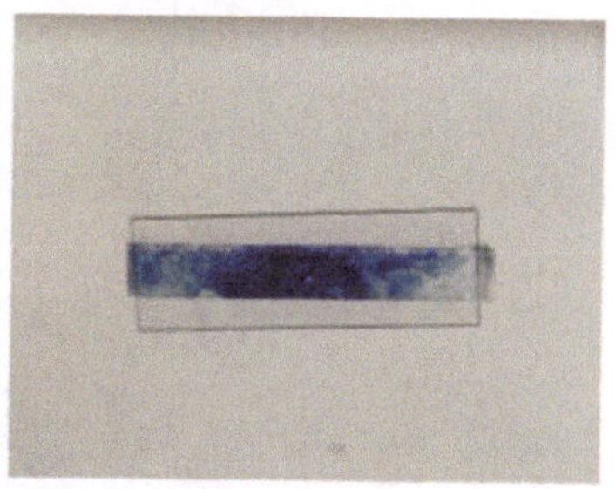

B

Figure 66: (A) Showing Acetate tape test **(B).** Acetate tape stained as glass slide.

Impression Smear and Swab Smear Examination

Impression or swab smears are generally made from the surface of suppurative or exudative skin lesions to differentiate between bacterial infection and sterile lesions such as in *Phemigus foliaceus*. The test is conducted by pressing the glass slide against the moist lesion, fixing it and then staining it. Alternatively a sterile swab can be used to collect purulent material. The swab is then rolled on the glass slide and processed further as in case of impression smear. The prepared slide is then examined microscopically. Different types of infections (Figure 67) can be identified.

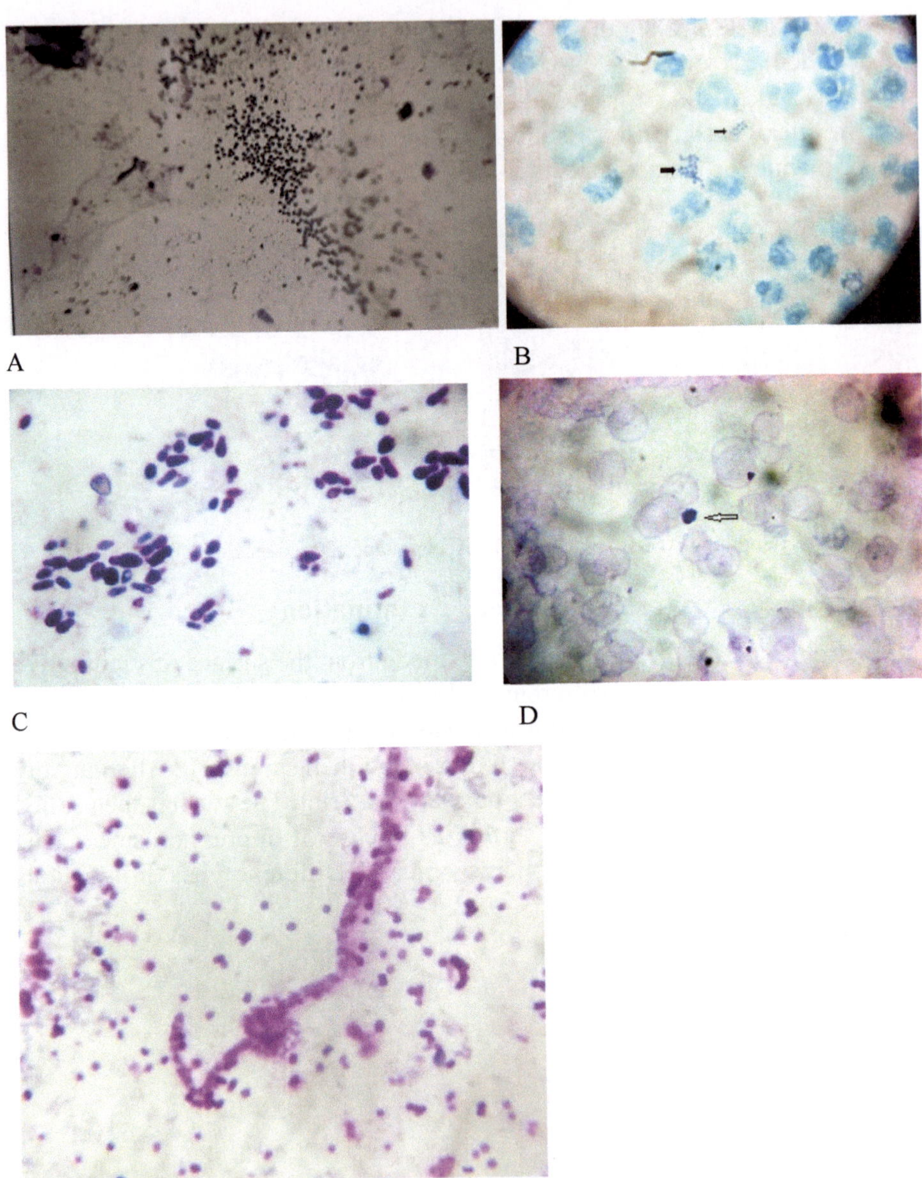

Figure 67: Impression smears showing organism **(A)** *S. aureus* in methylene blue stained smear **(B)**, *Malassezia pachydermatis* in methylene blue stained slide **(C)** Amastigote of *Leishmania* in Giemsa stained smear taken from lesion **(D)** and long chain Dermatophilus congolensis **(E)**.

Trichoscopy or Hair Plucks

It is rapid and inexpensive test for identifying demodex especially in foot area where skin scrapping is difficult. Area from where hairs are to be plucked, selected on the basis of dermatological examination. Hairs are generally plucked from the periphery of the lesion using tweezers (Figure 68), placed in a drop of liquid paraffin on the slide, covered with a cover slip and examined under microscope. *Demodex* mites are detected in association with the hair shaft (Figure68 B). Deep skin scrapping can be avoided. *Cheyletiella* mite or its cocooned eggs can also be detected by hair pluck technique. Follicular casts, hair damage due to dermatophytosis and evidence of keratinization can also be identified. This technique is being preferred over the skin scraping because of almost similar results but less invasive or traumatic. Microscopic examination of hair shaft (Figure 69) can provide evidence of mite infestations, dermatophyte infections, dysplastic hairs, and sometimes genetic diseases of hair coat.

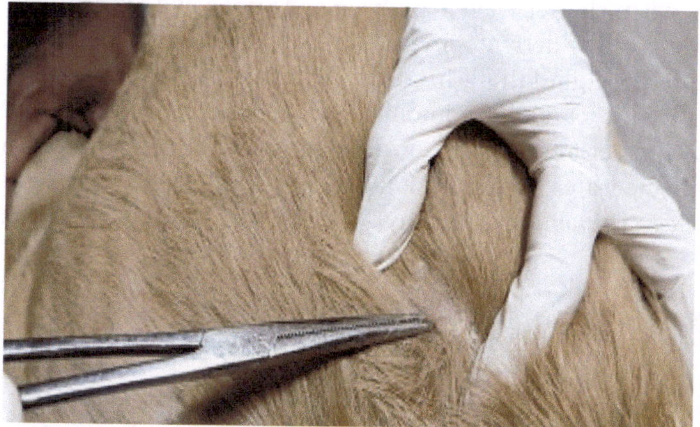

Figure 68: Showing plucking of the hairs from the periphery of the lesion.

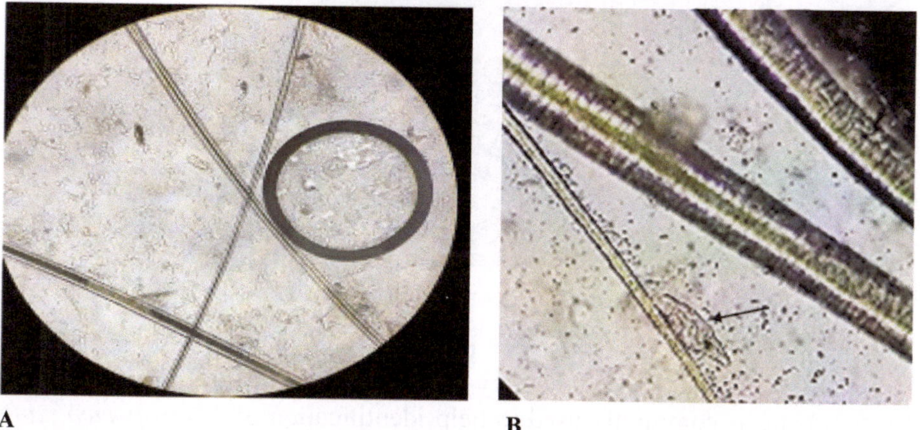

A B

Figure 69: **(A)** Showing microscopic examination of hair shaft. **(B)** Demodex is seen in association with hair shaft marked with arrow.

Wood's Lamp Examination

Wood's Lamp examination is a simple, easy, quick, painless and non-invasive technique available with clinician to assist diagnosis of certain type of fungal infection of the skin. The lamp was developed by an American physicist Robert Wood in 1903 and therefore named after him as Wood's Lamp or Wood's Light.

Wood's lamp (Figure 70) emits long wave ultraviolet light (320-450 nm, peak of 365 nm) through a nickel or cobalt glass filter and is employed to detect fluorescence in skin and hair. Emission of Wood's lamp long wave UV radiation is generated by a high pressure mercury arc fitted with a compound filter made of barium silicate and 9% nickel oxide. The filter is opaque to all lights except for a band between 320 and 450 nm with a peak of 365 nm.

Fluorescence occurs when shorter wave lengths are absorbed and longer wave length is emitted. Some of the dermatophytes exhibit fluorescence under long wave ultraviolet light. The light falling from the Wood's Lamp on the healthy skin usually appear purple or violet without any fluorescence. In the event of dermal infection with certain bacteria, or dermatophyte; or change in skin pigmentation, the affected area of skin changes color under ultraviolet light and show fluorescence. The area invaded by *M. canis* glow yellowish green (apple green).

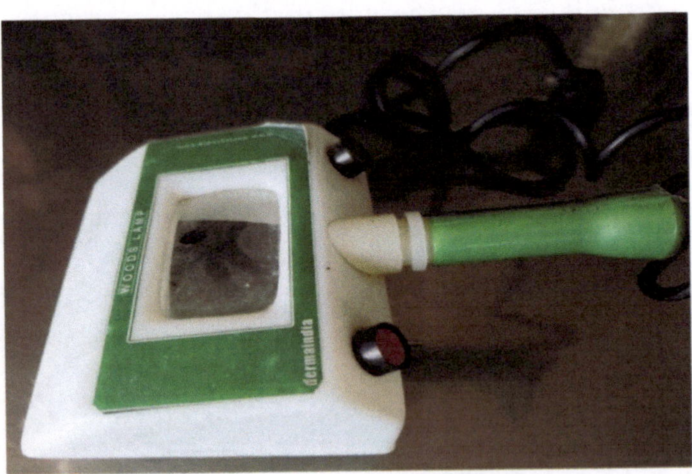

Figure 70: Showing Wood's Lamp.

In humans Wood's lamp is used to detect dermatophyte infection, bacterial infection, porphyria, and pigmentary diseases. In canine and feline medicine Wood's lamp is commonly used to help identification of *Microsporum canis* dermal infection. The metabolites of *Trichophyton* spp. and *Microsporum gypseum* do not cause fluorescence. Tryptophan is a metabolite of *M. canis that* causes fluorescence under ultraviolet light of 330-365 nm.

It is a complementary diagnostic aid. Fungal culture and/ or microscopic detection of arthrospores on hairs (Figure 71) is essential for confirmatory diagnosis. Fungal culture is more sensitive diagnostic test and is required for species identification. All strains of *M. canis* do not fluoresce. Only 30-80% strains of *M. canis* give fluorescence. Soap residue and seborrheic material may fluoresce. But that may not be apple green/emerald green of *M. canis*. Application of iodine destroys fluorescence. Only actively infected growing hairs fluorescence.

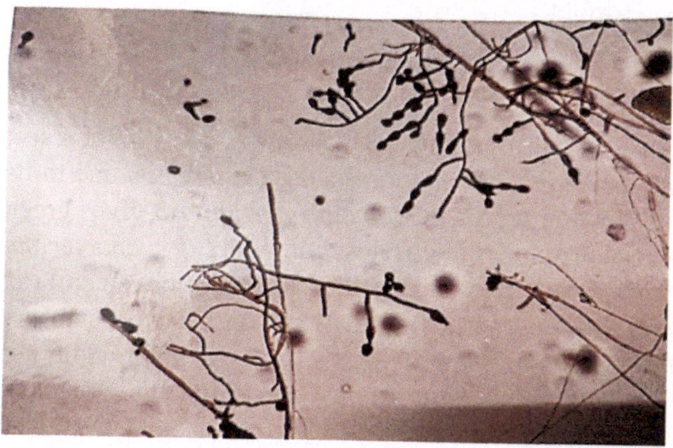

Figure 71: Culture and microscopic examination showing *Trichophyton* spp. Culture examination is essential for confirmation of species of fungus in skin infection.

It is desirable that the area to be examined under Wood's lamp should not have recently been washed or applied any medicine. Wet hairs /skin decreases the fluorescence. Contaminants such as detergents, fibers, soaps, serum, saliva, milk, wax, ointments produce false positive results. The Wood's lamp is turned on to warm up for about a minute or so. Some author recommends 20 seconds warm up. Room lights are turned off, and all doors and windows should remain closed to darken the surroundings completely. After adapting to the darkness, the skin is examined with Wood lamp for a few seconds (Figure 72). The lamp is held close to the hair coat (2-4 cm) to minimize false fluorescence. The examination is painless and safe. Turn off the Wood's lamp. Then turn on the lights of the room.

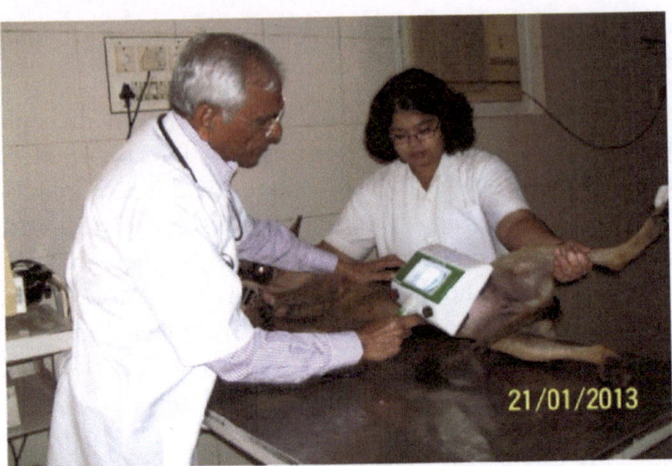

Figure 72: A dog is being examined under Wood's Lamp

Only infected hairs fluoresce. Surrounding skin or scales do not fluoresce. *Microsporum canis* gives yellowish green fluorescence (Figure 73) due to its metabolite tryptophane. Infection with *Pseudomonas aeruginosa* gives green fluorescence due to its secretion pyoverdine, a phosphor. With *Corynebacterium minutissimum*, causing superficial infection, erythrasma, fluoresces a coral red color owing to production of coproporphyrin III. Dust on hair coat appears blue-white. Thus negative results following Wood's lamp examination do not rule out dermatophytosis. Observation of the fluorescence should be confirmed by microscopic examination of the hairs.

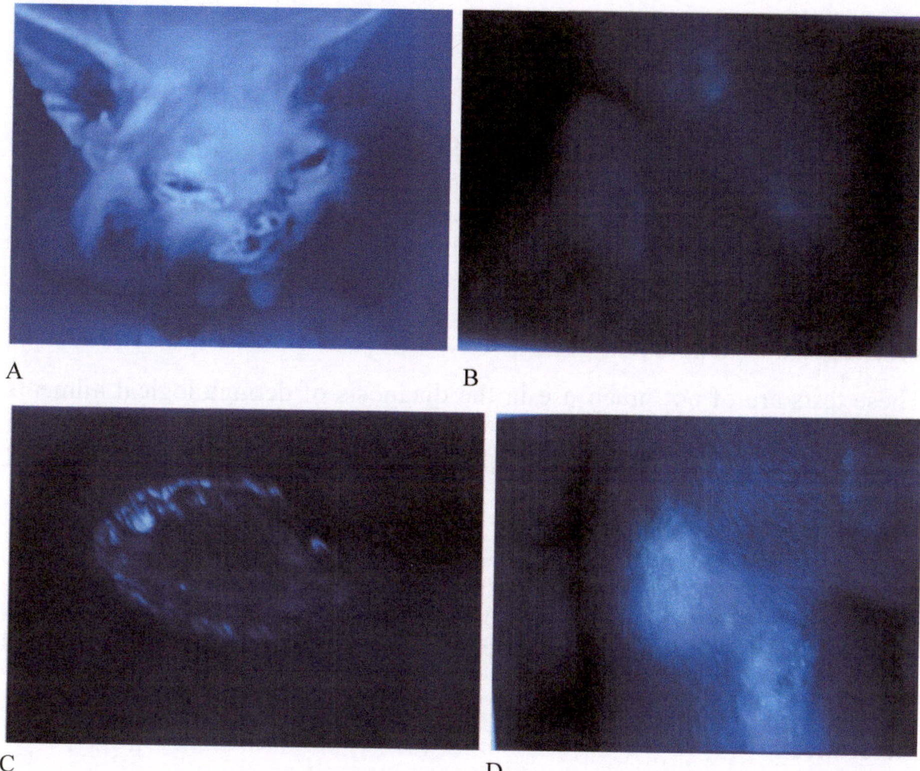

Figure 73: Skin lesions of cat **(A)** and dogs **(B, C and D)** showing yellowish green fluoresence suggesting *Microsporum canis* infection.

It is preferable to turn on the lamp for a few minutes before examining the patient to ensure stabilization of temperature dependent wave length. Sometimes infected hairs may require several minutes' exposure to the lamp light to start fluorescence. So short exposures may lead to false negative result. Scales, some topical applications and certain bacteria (*Pseudomonas aeruginosa* and *Corynebacterium minutissimum)* may have a greenish hue causing confusion and false positive result.

Culture Examination

Sterile swab samples, collected under ascetic conditions, are examined for bacterial and/or fungal culture and drug sensitivity. These samples are not refrigerated and shipped over night to lab. Cultural examination is indicated in skin infections unresponsive to treatment.

Biopsy and Histopathology

Biopsy is recommended when the lesion appears unusual and refractory to treatment. Biopsy is taken from an early active lesion. Punch biopsies (6-8 mm diameter) are used for intradermal lesion, and wedge biopsies are indicated for large nodular and subcutaneous lesions. Superficial lesion need not be scrubbed. Biopsy site is closed using 3-0 Vicryl or PDS. Biopsy samples are placed immediately in 10 % formalin solution and are sent to pathology laboratory for histopathological examination.

Routine Blood and Urine tests

These tests are of not much use in the diagnosis of dermatological ailments unless systemic signs of illness are associated. In recurrent dermatological problems, these tests may be helpful in identifying underlying subclinical disease.

Intradermal testing

Intradermal testing is done to identify an allergen in cases of atopic dermatitis. In vitro tests (ELISA or RAST) are becoming an alternative to intradermal tests.

Reference

Varshney, J.P.(2023). Heart Failure in Animals: Current Concept. NIPA® GENX Electronic Resources & Solutions P. LTD. New Delhi-110 034.

9

Clinical Diagnostic Techniques in Otology

Otology is the branch of medicine concerned with the study of the ear and its diseases. Ear diseases in canines have multiple etiology varying from allergies (food or environmental), ectoparasites, infections (bacteria, malassazia, fungus), endocrine disorders, immunological disorders (autoimmune diseases), foreign material, neoplasms to keratinization disorders. For rational management, correct diagnosis is a pre-requisite. Diagnostic techniques in otology include history, clinical examination including ear canal palpation and visual inspection of ears, imaging (otoscopy, radiography, CT scan, MRI, and ultrasonography) and cytological evaluation of otic contents/ discharge.

History and Clinical Examination

Like other organs of the body, a thorough analysis of history and detail physical examination is imperative for diagnosing diseases of the ear. In case allergy is speculated as a cause of ear disease, diet elimination trial is to be considered before performing allergy testing. Otitis externa in senior dogs with no previous history of ear disease, requires consideration of systemic triggers with routine checkup for health profiles and endocrine function tests. Pinna (Figure 74) should be carefully examined for the presence of lesion. Superficial and deep scrapping should to taken for detection of mites.

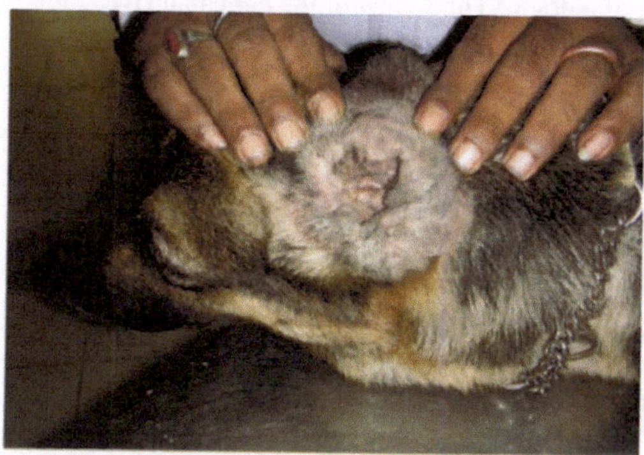

Figure 74: Examination of ear pinna showing thickening of skin lining

Imaging Techniques

Otoscopy, radiography, computed tomography, magnetic resonance imaging and ultrasonography are the imaging techniques being used in the diagnosis of ear diseases.

Otoscopy (Figure 75), a technique of diagnostic imaging, is a method of choice to examine the external ear canal as well as to identify an existing otitis media and examination of wall of the canal. It is a part of minimum data base. The technique is helpful in identification of canal proliferation, masses, foreign bodies, ruptured tympanic membrane, changes in integrity and density of tympanic membrane, large bulging pars flaccida, suggesting primary secretory otitis media seen in cavalier King Charles spaniels (Cole, 2012). Any as discharge) from ear (Figure 76) should be collected and examined. Samples for investigation are to be collected from the pinna, and ear canal as the case may be for cytology. Ear canal assessment for chronic change is to be done prior to otoscopic examination. Alteration (reduction) in lumen and calcification of the canals can be determined by palpation.

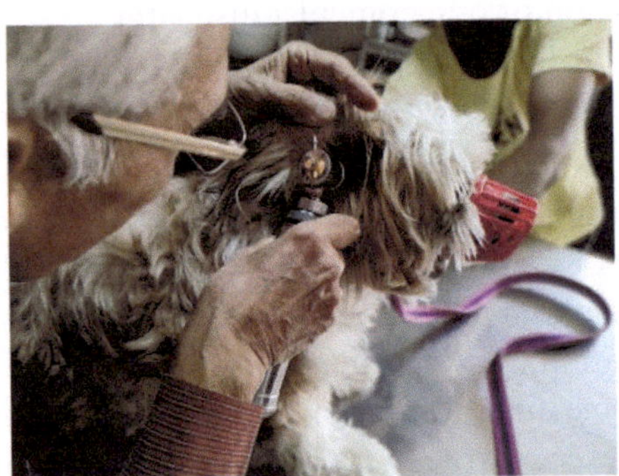

A

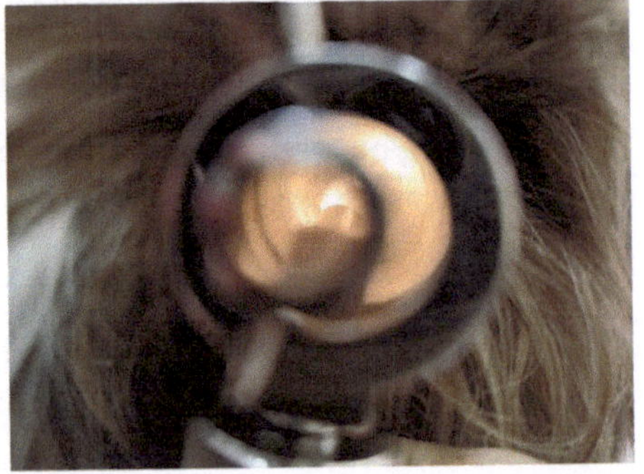

B

Figure 75: Showing otoscopic examination of a dog **(A)** and view of the ear canal **(B)**.

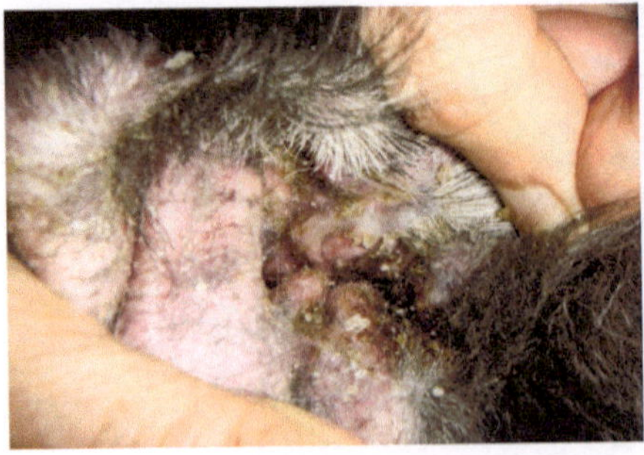

Figure 76: Showing crust, thickening and thick discharge from ear.

Radiographic examination is valuable in the evaluation of the osseous tympanic bulla and the external ear canals (for mineralization or stenosis). It has limited value in detecting soft tissue changes especially in acute cases. General anesthesia is indicated for right positioning to take radiographs to evaluate the tympanic bulla. Radiograph should be taken in three most common views (dorso-ventral, rostrocaudal and lateral oblique).

Computed tomography and magnetic resonance imaging (MRI) are far better than radiography for visualization of middle ear. These techniques are used to evaluate communication of fistulous tracts and abscesses with the external ear canal. These techniques can assist in the early diagnosis of the subtle abnormalities. Computed tomography aids in differentiation of bony lesions in the bullae from soft tissue reactions. MRI aids in visualizing middle and inner ear and detects presence of fluids, such as endolymph within the cochlea and semicircular canals.

Ultrasonography is another diagnostic technique that can detect fluid within the tympanic bullae.

Brainstem-evoked Auditory Responses

The technique is used to measure hearing in dogs with otitis.

Ear canal Cytology

Cytological examination (Figure 77) of ear canal discharge is an important diagnostic technique that provides information about aural environment and infection. It is the primary diagnostic tool in identifying bacterial or yeast overgrowth. Cytological examination should be performed prior to bacteriological culture and antibiotic sensitivity because it may not be required if there is yeast overgrowth.

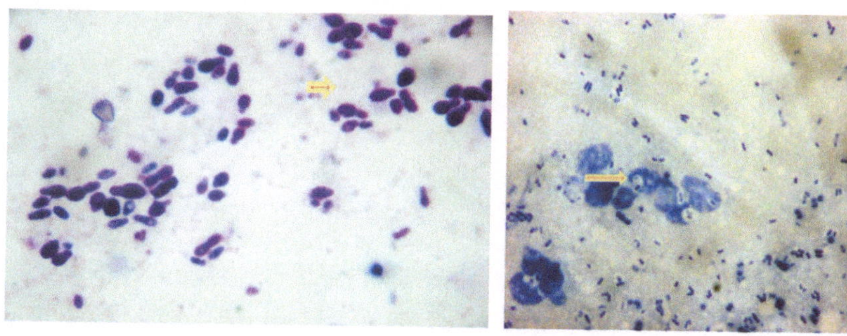

A B

Figure 77: Cytological examination of ear exudate showing preponderance of Malassazia (A) and preponderance of Gram -ve bacilli and presence of bacilli in phagocytes.

Reference

Cole, L.K. (2012).Primary secretory otitis media in Cavalier King Charles Spaniels. Vet. Clin. Small Anim .Pract. N. Am. 42:1137-1142.

10

Clinical Diagnostic Techniques in Gastro-Enterology

Diseases of gastro-intestinal tract are very common in dogs and cats. Gastro-intestinal tract starts from mouth to anus. The first step in making diagnosis of gastro-intestinal disease is to localize the problem. Whether it is buccal cavity, esophagus, stomach, or intestines. Cursory history for seemingly simple complaint like vomiting, anorexia or loose feces may be unrewarding because gastrointestinal diseases may be primary (concerning with only gastro-intestinal tract and its functions) or secondary (due to underlying disease/disorder of organs other than gastro-intestinal tract). Therefore, for ascertaining the cause of gastrointestinal signs (anorexia, nausea, vomiting, regurgitation, constipation, loose feces, bloody feces), a thorough examination of all body systems is more logical. As with other body systems, a comprehensive systematic approach is needed for diagnosing diseases of gastro-intestinal tract also. The techniques for the diagnosis of gastro-intestinal diseases include examination of history, physical examination, urine examination, fecal examination, pancreatic function tests, intestinal function tests, application of imaging tools (radiography, ultrasonography, and endoscopy) and cytology or histopathology.

History

Detail history regarding day to day eating and elimination habits, type of food being fed, change in food if any, water intake, urination, deworming status, vaccination status, weight loss/gain, vomiting/regurgitation, constipation/diarrhea and any change in behavior should be obtained. Signalment details should invariably be recorded. History with respect to diet (treats, table food, supplementation of vitamins and or calcium, flavored food, food with corn or wheat), frequency (how many times a day) and amount of feed being offered is of diagnostic concern.

Physical Examination

Next important step is to localize the problem and distinguishing between vomiting and regurgitation; and between small and large intestine diarrhea. Examination with respect to posture, behavior, attitude, vital signs (temperature, respiration, pulse), hydration status (skin turgidity, capillary refill time, color of mucus membrane), body condition score and abdominal status should be conducted. Distended abdomen may be due to ascites, tumor, hepato or splenomegaly, gas accumulation, gastric dilatation/ volvulus. Salivation and lip smacking may be suggestive of nausea, gastric or esophageal reflex or hepatic encephalopathy. Regurgitation (megaesophagus, esophageal stenosis, gastric motility disorder), excessive salivation (foreign body in dogs, hepatic encephalopathy in cats), oral ulceration (CRF), and halitosis (dental disease, foreign body) are suggestive of abnormalities related to upper gastro-intestinal tract. Increased borborygmus are suggestive of enteritis or inflammatory bowel disease (lower gastrointestinal tract). Large volume diarrhea indicates involvement of small intestines while small volume diarrhea suggests large intestines' involvement. Similarly, melena suggests hemorrhage/ bleeding in upper gastrointestinal tract and fresh frank blood in feces suggests its origin from lower gastrointestinal tract. Palpation of abdomen and rectal palpation should be done as a part of clinical examination.

Urine Analysis

It may provide an overall assessment of health and also inclusion or exclusion of some diseases (kidney disease, urinary tract infection, diabetes). Low volume of urine may be due to fever or dehydration.

Fecal Examination

Feces are routinely subjected to direct examination (color, consistency, stickiness, mucus, coccidian oocysts or Giardia trophozoites), parasitological examination (presence of parasitic ova, cysts) and cytological examination (for organisms) .Colorless or pale (acholic) feces are seen in bile duct obstruction or in exocrine pancreatic insufficiency. Melena (tarry or black feces) indicates hemorrhage/ ulcer in upper gastro-intestinal tract. Fresh blood in feces may be due to hemorrhage in lower gastrointestinal tract or parasites. Feces should also be looked for the presence of foreign material if any. Greasy feces suggests mal absorption syndrome (protein -losing enteropathy) or exocrine pancreatic insufficiency. *Giardia* trophozoites and coccidian oocysts can be detected on direct microscopic examination of feces. Fecal examination using flotation and zinc sulfate centrifugation technique should be done for identification of parasitic ova to ruled out or ruled in parasitism as a cause of diarrhea. Fecal cytology is recommended for identifying cells (neutrophils, eosinophils), spores of *Clostridium* (safety pin shaped), *Campylobacter, Cryptosporidium*, Mycobacteria or fungal infection (Histoplasma).

Giardia antigen test (if direct test for Giardia is negative), Parvo virus antigen test and fecal culture (for *Salmonella, Campylobacter, E. coli*) tests can also be conducted in puppies with diarrhea and vomiting.

In exocrine pancreatic insufficiency feces are voluminous and rancid; undigested striated muscle fibers are detected microscopically in new methylene blue stained fecal slides (Figure78); X-ray film strip incubated with a mixture of fresh feces and sodium bicarbonate for 60 minutes at 37°C remains undigested (Figure79); and feces stained with Lugol's iodine (2%) reveals predominance of blue-black granules (Figure 80). Detection of undigested fat in feces, decreased proteases activity (presence of striated muscle fibers and no digestion of x-ray film) and decreased amylase activity in feces (no digestion of x-ray film) lend support to the presumptive diagnosis of exocrine pancreatic insufficiency (Bunch, 1992).

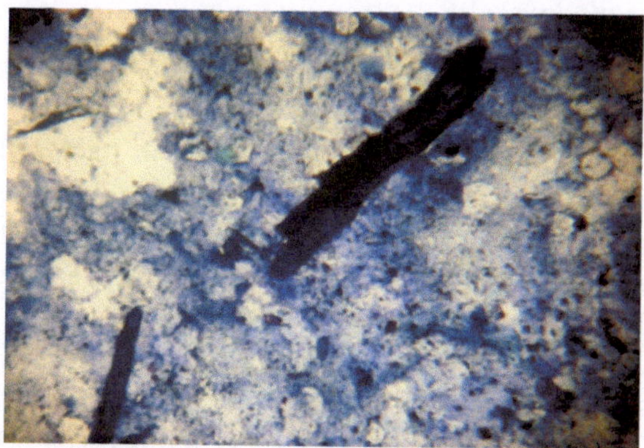

Figure 78: Feces stained with New Methylene Blue showing striated muscle fibers.

Figure 79: X-Ray film incubated with feces remained undigested.

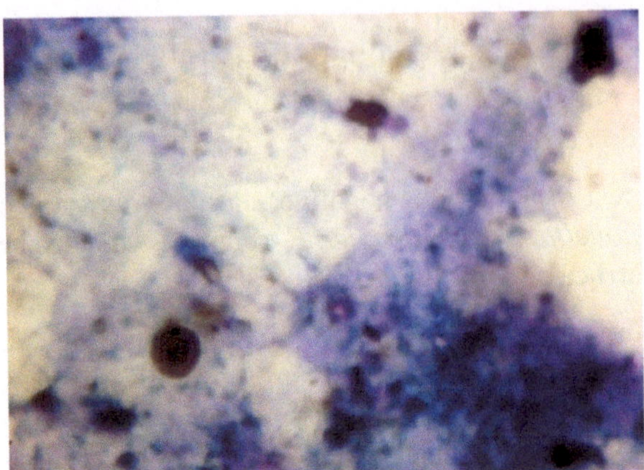

Figure 80: Feces stained with Lugol's showing preponderance of blue black granules.

Pancreatic Function Tests

Serum lipase, amylase and serum trypsin like immunoreactivity (TLI) tests are conducted for evaluating pancreas function. Canine pancreatic elastase has also shown promise in the diagnosis of acute pancreatitis.

Intestinal Function Tests

Serum level of cobalamin (B12) decreases and folate increases in bacterial overgrowth or exocrine pancreatic insufficiency. Low level of folate is indicative of upper small intestine diseases and low level of cobalamin is indicative of lower small intestine disease. Low levels of both folate and cobalamin are seen when entire small intestine is affected.

Cytology

Pancreatic cytology or histopathology provides definite diagnosis of pancreatitis or pancreatic tumor.

Radiography

In cases of acute and severe vomiting, radiography can be of immense value in ruling out or ruling in foreign bodies (Figure81), gastric distension (Figure82), gastric dilatation /volvulus (Figure83), intussusception, or tumors. Contrast radiography may be valuable assist in detecting large hemorrhaging/perforating ulcers, esophageal stenosis, mega-esophagus (Figure84), diaphragmatic hernia (Figure85), paralytic ileus (Figure86). Abdominal radiography is of limited value in cases of chronic gastro-intestinal problems.

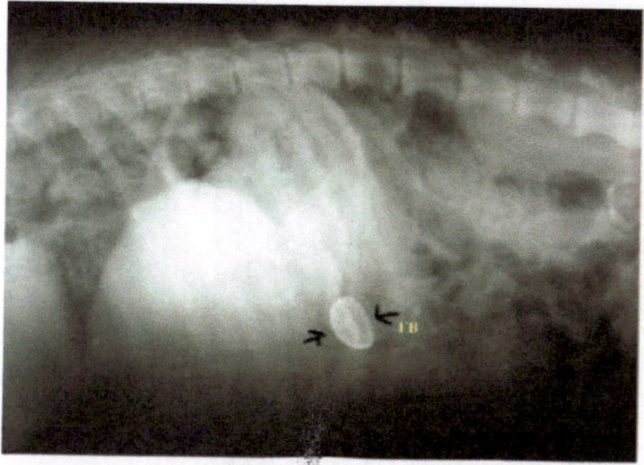

Figure 81: Abdominal radiograph of a dog showing foreign body in stomach.

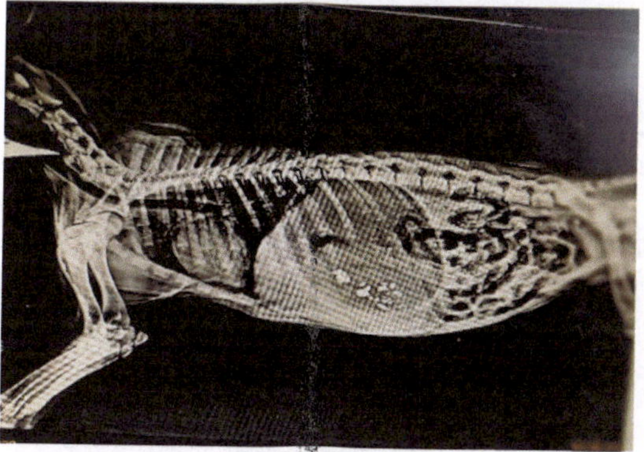

Figure 82: Abdominal radiograph of a dog showing gastric distension.

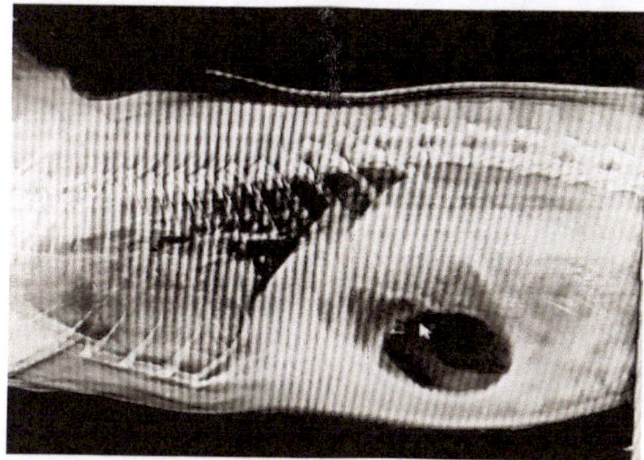

Figure 83: Abdominal radiograph of a dog showing gastric dilatation and volvulus

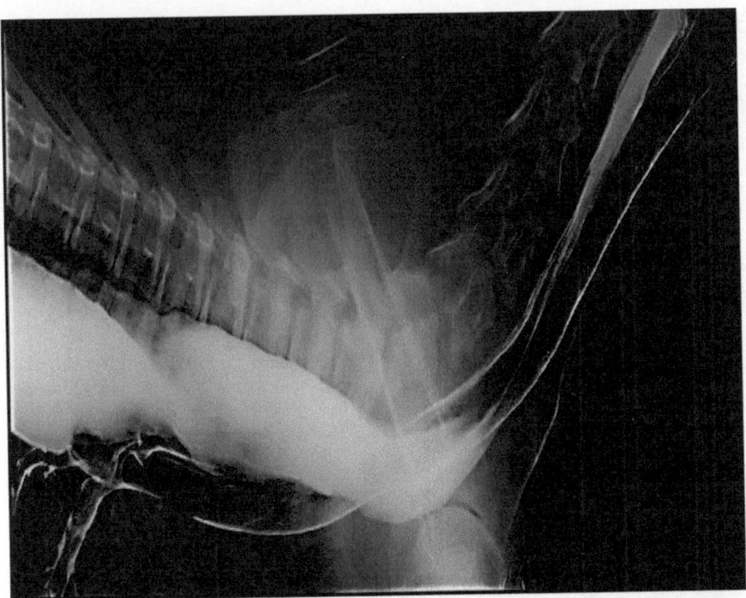

Figure 84: Contrast radiograph (barium meal) of a dog showing mega-esophagus

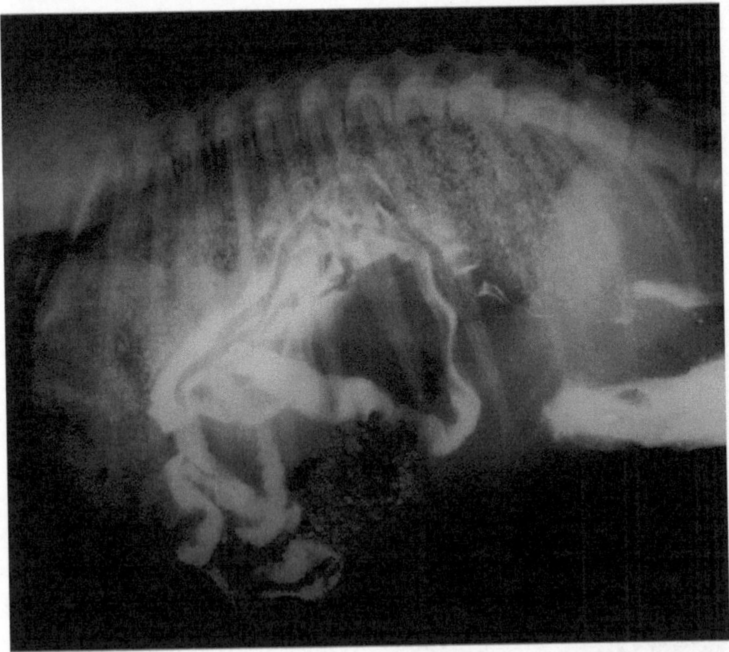

Figure 85: Contrast radiograph of a dog showing diaphragmatic hernia

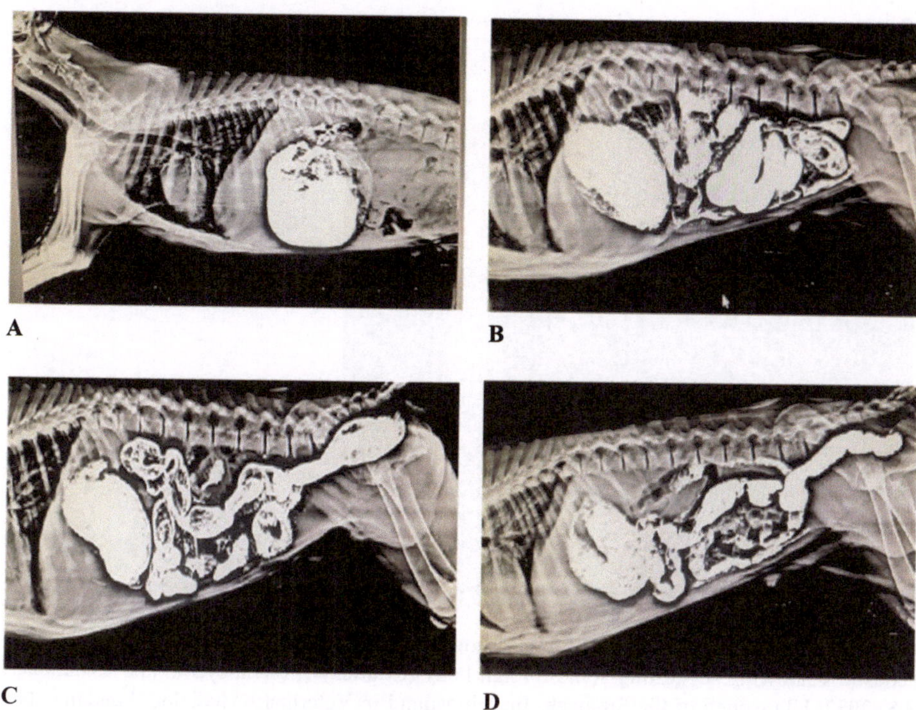

Figure 86: Contrast radiographs of a five month old non-descript male pup weighing 6.1 kg with persistant vomiting, no passage of feces and anorexia for four days showing retension of barium in gastrointestinal tract even up to 72 hrs (**A** –immediate after barium meal, **B**- 24 hrs after barium meal, **C**- 48 hrs after barium meal and **D**- 72 hrs after barium meal) suggesting adymanic ileus or paralytic ileus.

Abdominal Ultrasonography

Abdominal ultrasonography is a valuable diagnostic test in detecting gastric ulceration, gastric masses, gastric foreign bodies (Figure87), gastritis, intussusception (Figure88), intestinal foreign bodies, intestinal perforation, intestinal masses, and enlargement of mesenteric lymph nodes. Normal pancreas is not visible in ultrasound, but diseased pancreas can be visualized. Pancreas enlargement and fluid around pancreas with change in pancreatic echogenicity is suggestive of pancreatitis and necrosis.

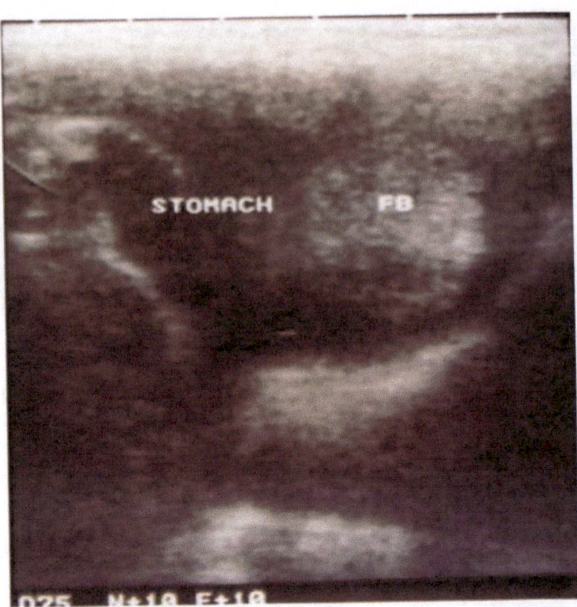

Figure 87: Abdominal sonogram of a dog showing irregular shaped material in stomach with acoustic shadowing suggesting some foreign body (Courtesy : Varshney,J.P. and Chaudhary, P.S. 2022. Ultrasound of the Stomach. In: Ultrasound in Veterinary Medicine. Fundamentals and Applications. NIPA GENX Electronic Resources and Solutions P.Ltd. New Delhi-110 034).

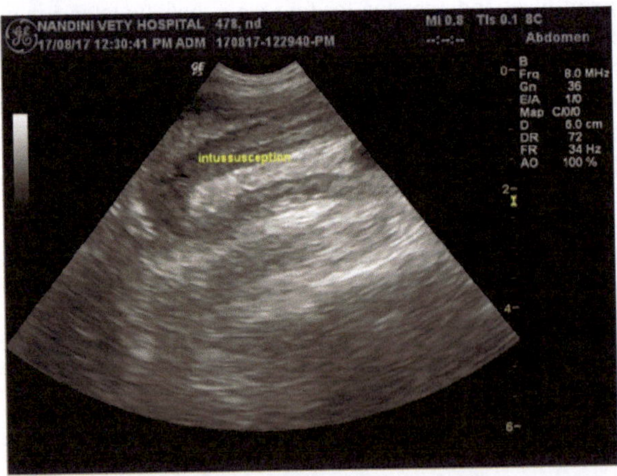

Figure 88: Transabdominal sonograms of a dog showing multilayered appearance in longitudinal axis suggesting intestinal intussusception (Courtesy : Varshney, J.P. and Chaudhary, P.S. 2022. Ultrasound of the Intestines. In: Ultrasound in Veterinary Medicine. Fundamentals and Applications. NIPA GENX Electronic Resources and Solutions P.Ltd. New Delhi- 110 034).

Gastroscopy and Endoscopy

Gastroscopy and endoscopy/ laparoscopy (Figure89) techniques are valuable in localizing disease in suspected cases of gastrointestinal disease (generalized gastro-intestinal disease, disease of stomach, disease of duodenum or disease of colon) to localize the lesion. The endoscopic techniques can also assist in taking biopsy. An insertion of laparoscope and laparoscopic view of the liver of a dog revealing cobbler stone appearance is shown in Figure90.

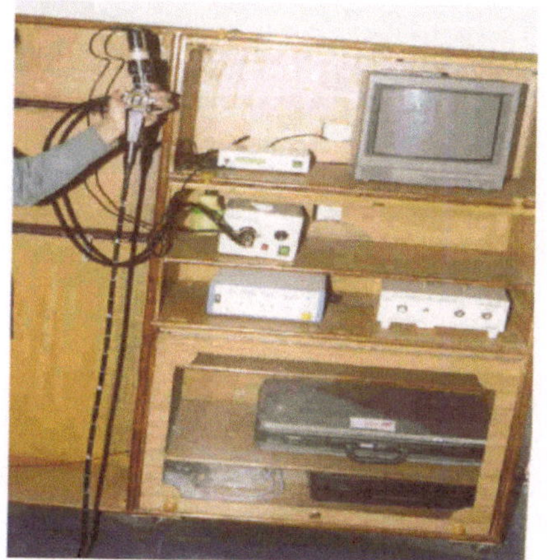

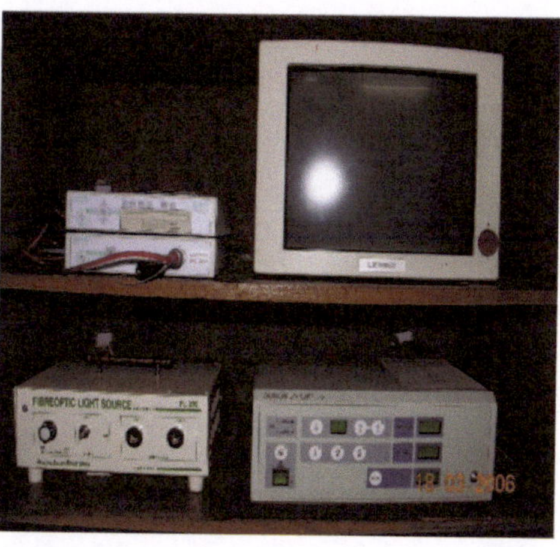

A B

Figure 89: Showing Gastroscope **(A)** and Laparoscope **(B)**

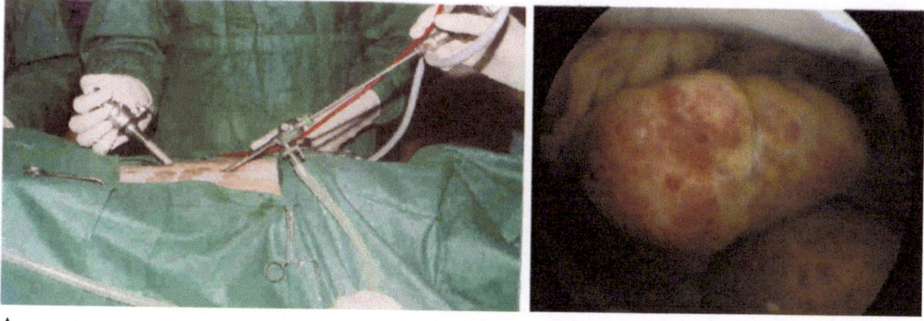

A **B**

Figure 90: Showing insertion of laparoscope **(A)** and laparoscopic view of the liver revealing cobblerstone appearance of the liver **(B)**.

Reference

Bunch, S.E. (1992) : Diseases of the Exocrine Pancreas. In : Handbook of Small Animal Practice. Morgan, R.V. (ed). W.B. Saunders Company, Philadelphia, pp. 459 – 471.

11

Clinical Diagnostic Techniques in Hepatology

The term "Hepatology" is derived from the Greek words "hepatikos" and "logia" meaning liver and study respectively. It is the branch of medicine dealing with the study of structure, function, diseases and abnormalities of the liver, gall bladder, and biliary tree. Liver/hepatic diseases in companion pets vary from multifactorial hepatitis (acute and chronic), cirrhosis, portosystemic shunt, copper storage disease, hepatic lipidosis, and hepatic neoplasm to fulminant hepatic failure. The etiology of liver diseases also varies from infection, auto-immune, metabolic to genetic factors. The hepatic disorders are quite common in canines and felines. Moreover, the diagnosis of liver malfunctioning is loosely given in pet practice without any supportive evidence. Diagnosing specific liver disease is a challenging task as the symptoms of hepatic diseases are ambiguous with delayed expression. Many cases may not show any symptom despite existing severely damaged liver. Sometimes it may be frustrating as liver enzymes (heavy reliance paid by practitioners) and other biochemical indices indicate liver dysfunction but fail to identify the type of liver pathology. Changes in some of the liver enzymes (ALT, SAP) is also seen in diseases of other organs. Even ultrasonography alone does not specify liver disease except reflecting echogenic changes. Ultrasonography is of diagnostic value in gall bladder diseases. Radiography is mostly restricted to reveal the liver size. Clinical manifestations of hepatic disorders are vague and are seen in many other diseases. In view of these facts diagnosis of hepatobiliary diseases poses a challenge .Therefore, a comprehensive systematic approach is needed for the correct diagnosis of liver diseases, A systematic approach for diagnosing liver disorders comprises of various techniques such as examination of history, detail clinical examination, hepatic enzymes (ALT, SAP, GGT), biomarkers (Kallistatin), biochemical panel (blood glucose, serum proteins with A/G ratio,, bilirubin, cholesterol, bile acid etc.), hepatic imaging (plain abdominal radiography, hepatic ultrasound, CT scan and MRI), biopsy, hemogram, and urine examination as per the requirement of the case.

History

A proper history is pre-requisite to define and identify clinically relevant problems to be addressed. Liver has tremendous reserve capacity (80%) and potential to regenerate. Symptoms of liver failure appear when liver reserves are exhausted. Because of liver reserves, the overt clinical manifestations are prevented. As a result, the disease remains sub clinical for a petty long time. Nevertheless, history of mild increase in frequency of drinking water and urination, weakness, lethargy and recurrent vomiting appears suggestive of impending liver disorder.

Clinical Manifestations

Anorexia, weakness, vomiting, light colored or black tarry faces, dullness, depression, diarrhea, fever, abdominal pain, weight loss, polydipsia, polyuria, abdominal distension (Figure 91), icterus (Figure 91), seizures, neurological signs, itching, change in liver size, dark colored urine and coma are the clinical manifestations observed in liver diseases. These manifestations are non-specific and ambiguous. Therefore, diagnosis of liver diseases cannot exactly be ascertained solely on the basis of clinical symptoms alone. Nevertheless, the clinical signs may provide clue for further investigations.

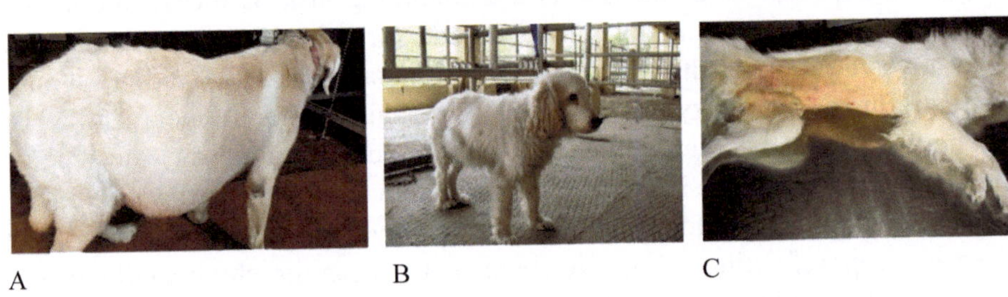

A B C

Figure 91: Showing abdominal distension **(A, B)** and icteric body © in dogs later diagnosed with cirrhosis **(A and B)** and biliary obstruction © on detail investigations.

Hepatic Enzymology

(i) Alanine aminotransferase (ALT or SGPT) is a liver specific enzyme in dogs and cats. Its half-life is < 24 hrs. Its concentration is increased following severe, acute and diffuse hepatocellular necrosis. Peak level of ALT is attained after 48-72 hrs. of hepatic insult. Two-to-three-fold increase in the level of the ALT is considered significant suggestive of pathology. Increase in ALT level has also been seen in non- hepatic diseases (inflammatory disease of gastrointestinal tract such as pancreatitis and inflammatory bowel disease, hemolytic anemia or cardiac failure) and in patients on anticonvulsant or glucocorticoid therapy. ALT level also increases in biliary stasis, endocrinopathies (diabetes mellitus, hyperadrenocorticism), and status epilepticus,

(ii) Alkaline phosphatase (ALP) is an enzyme bound to membranes of bile canaliculi and bile ducts. The enzyme is released in conditions causing intra or extra hepatic cholestasis. Isoenzymes of alkaline phosphatase are also found in bone, intestine, kidneys and placenta. Isoenzymes found in kidneys, placenta and intestines has a very short life as compared to those found in liver and bones. Exogenous and endogenous glucocorticoids also cause an increase in the level of specific isoenzyme of ALP in dogs. Increased level of ALP is also seen in young growing pups; in dogs with degenerative bone disease, certain carcinomas and mammary gland tumors; and in dogs receiving anticonvulsant therapy.

These enzymes (ALT and ALP) cannot ascertain whether the dog is having hepatic or post hepatic disease as an increase is observed in both conditions. Definite correlation between the magnitude of enzyme increases and severity of the disease is lacking as there is minimum or no increase in severe hepatic dysfunction associated with liver cirrhosis, liver neoplasm, portacaval shunt or intrahepatic portal shunts.

(iii) Gamma glutamyl transpeptidase (GGT) is another enzyme found in the liver and an increase in its level is seen in almost all conditions in which ALP level increases except in pups with an increased osteoblastic activity and in dogs on anticonvulsant therapy.

New Biomarker

Kallistatin is mainly synthesized and secreted in the liver. Its average concentration is reduced significantly in patients with liver cirrhosis of different etiologies. It is a new and reliable biomarker for the diagnosis of hepatic cirrhosis. It is a protein produced by SERPINA 4 gene. A close correlation has been observed between reduction in serum kallistatin levels and severity of early hepatic disease.

Biochemical Indicators

(a) *Serum Proteins*

Liver plays a vital role in protein metabolism. Albumin is exclusively synthesized in the liver and it contributes to total serum/plasma proteins. The liver has a large reserve capacity for the synthesis of albumin and it has a serum half-life of approximately 7 days in dogs (Lakner,2011). Synthesis of the albumin is affected because of reduced functional ability of the liver owing to severe hepatic disease. Because of tremendous hepatic reserve, hypoalbuminemia occurs at a loss of around 70-80% liver function. Measurement of plasma/ serum proteins, albumin and prothrombin time can be used to assess the liver function. Prolonged prothrombin time is a specific indicator of impaired synthetic capacity of the liver. Hypoalbuminemia has been reported in cirrhosis, portosystemic encephalopathy and in severe diffuse necrosis. A decrease in albumin concentrations has also been recorded in renal and gut disease, severe cutaneous burns, protein malnutrition, in the presence of acute phase reactants, and in patients with exudative effusions. Therefore hypoalbuminemia is insensitive marker for hepatic insufficiency and is only evident in cases with advanced chronic liver disease or portosystemic shunts (Xenoulis and Steiner, 2011 and Lakner *et al.*, 2011). Globulins are not exclusively produced by the liver. Liver produces α (alpha) and β (beta) globulins. Gamma (γ) globulins are produced by lymphoid cells. An increase in serum globulin level may occur in inflammatory hepatic disease or in compromised hepatic reticuloendothelial system. Hepatic insufficiency rarely leads to a decrease in serum globulin concentration (Lakner *et al.*,2011). A decrease in globulin level may be seen in dogs with portosystemic encephalopathy.

Most of the coagulation factors are synthesized in the liver. Prothrombin and thromboplastin are important component of coagulation. Prothrombin time and activated partial thromboplastin time are prolonged in acute hepatic necrosis (Dunayer and Gwaltney-Brant, 2006). While in congenital portosystemic vascular problems only activated partial thromboplastin time is prolonged (Niles *et al.*,2001 and Kummeling *et al.*,2006).

Ammonia is produced in the intestines, carried to liver and is converted to blood urea nitrogen and excreted through kidneys. Liver function is compromised in portosystemic shunting affecting the metabolization of ammonia resulting into increased level of blood ammonia (hyperammonemia). Hyperammonemia facilitates the formation of ammonium biurate crystalluria that is commonly seen in dogs with portosystemic shunting. Hyperammonemia leads to hepatic encephalopathy. Increase in fasting plasma ammonia level seems reliable and notable indicator in dogs with portosystemic shunts. It is superior to fasting plasma bile acid (Gerritzen-Bruning *et al.*,2006).

(b) *Bilirubinaemia and Bilirubinuria*

Bilirubin is the breakdown product of heme containing compounds in the spleen that is carried to the liver where it is conjugated. Conjugated bilirubin (direct) is excreted into the bile and carried to intestine and is converted to urobilinogen and stercobilin. Mild bilirubinuria can occur in healthy dogs; in dogs during starvation and during fever. Level of total bilirubin varies with different disease processes. Its concentrations are higher in dogs with hemolytic disease (pre-hepatic) as compared to hepatic disease. Icteric signs are seen when bilirubin is exceeding 2.5-3.0 mg/dl. Total bilirubin has two fractions as unconjugated (indirect) and conjugated (direct) moieties. Conjugated bilirubin form covalent bond with albumin (bilirubin -protein complexes or delta bilirubin) and remains in circulation for sustained period. It is slowly catabolized leading to sustained icterus (one – two weeks). Increase in only conjugated bilirubin (direct)level is indicative of post hepatic jaundice (biliary tract obstruction or pancreatic disease). In hepatic jaundice both conjugated (direct) and unconjugated (indirect) bilirubin levels increase. In prehepatic jaundice unconjugated bilirubin increases. Unconjugated bilirubin concentration also increases in dogs with acquired portosystemic shunting. In dogs with sepsis, mild bilirubinemia and bilirubinuria may be noted. Bilirubinuria occurs well before jaundice is seen owing to low renal threshold. Studies have revealed no clinical utility of fractionation of bilirubin in healthy dogs, dogs with pre-hepatic (hemolytic) or hepatic jaundice. An increase in urinary urobilinogen can be ascribed to increase bilirubin production, decrease bilirubin clearance, or increase production by intestinal microorganisms. No urinary urobilinogen in icteric dog with acholic feces is suggestive of bile duct obstruction. Urinary urobilinogen has been used earlier to diagnose biliary patency. At present it is of not much clinical significance.

(c) *Cholesterol*

Cholesterol level may be affected in liver diseases. Congenital or acquired portosystemic shunt and fulminant liver failure may be associated with low level of serum cholesterol. In jaundiced cat with major bile duct obstruction, serum cholesterol concentration increases. Increase in serum cholesterol is also noted in non-hepatic diseases (pancreatitis, diabetes mellitus, hyperadrenocorticism and hypothyroidism).

(d)Bile acids

Serum bile acids are a sensitive screening test for hepatic encephalopathy and in dogs and cats. In some cases of hepatic neoplasia, normal level of bile acids has been reported. Though level of serum bile acid increases with the severity of the hepatobiliary disease, provides no information about the type of lesion or its reversibility. Concentration of serum bile acid is not influenced by steroids.

(e) Vitamin D

It is fat soluble sterol derivative predominantly synthesized in the liver and has multiple functions (Marolf,2016). There are some indications that clinical signs and prognosis of chronic liver diseases are associated with serum level of vitamin D. Reports indicate that there is a decrease in serum vitamin D level to the extent of insufficiency or deficiency in chronic liver diseases in humans. Reduction in vitamin D levels associated with chronic cholestatic liver disease in dogs can largely be due to secondary malabsorption of the vitamin D due to the absence of adequate amounts of bile salts in the intestinal lumen, or by other factors which seem independent of the hepatic metabolism of vitamin D (Plourde *et al.*,1988).

Imaging Techniques

(a) Abdominal Radiography

Plain routine abdominal radiographs may be helpful in confirming the size of the liver (large or small liver- Figure 92), asymmetric enlargement of a liver lobe or border margins of the liver (regular or irregular) and abdominal effusions (Figure 92). Because of large solid organ, plain film evaluation may not be rewarding. Mineralized densities overlying liver parenchyma or biliary structures can be suggestive of choleliths or dystrophic mineralization associated with congenital bile duct malformation. Air densities within hepatic parenchyma or biliary structures are suggestive of emphysematous process. Contrast radiography may be some help in diagnosing portacaval shunts. Contrast radiography of biliary system is not commonly used.

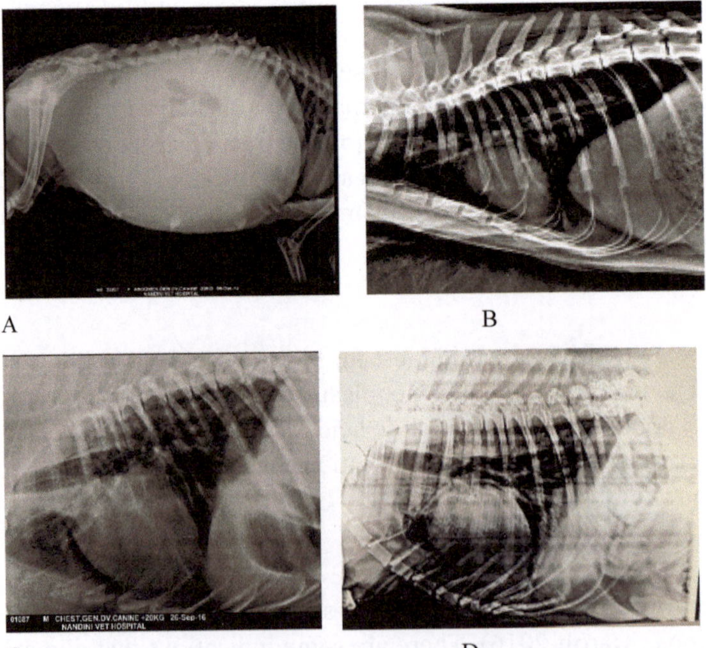

Figure 92: Radiographs of dogs showing peritoneal effusions **(A)**, liver of normal size **(B)**, liver of reduced size **(C)** and liver of large size protruding out of the rib cage **(D)**.

(b)Abdominal Ultrasonography

Hepatic ultrasound is a non-invasive diagnostic technique gaining momentum in the diagnosis of hepatic diseases (Figure93). Liver ultrasound has a potential of differentiating focal liver disease from the diffuse liver disease, cystic lesion from solid masses, and obstructive jaundice from non-obstructive jaundice. It has made the diagnosis of intra or extra hepatic portosystemic shunts and gall bladder diseases (cholecystitis, GB calculi, sludge, bile duct obstruction) possible that was otherwise speculative. Hepatic sonography is routinely indicated in dogs with increased or decreased hepatic enzymes, ascites, suspected with liver tumor/mass, detection of abdominal metastasis, congenital/ acquired portocaval or portosystemic shunt , biliary diseases, blood flow abnormalities (Doppler ultrasound) and for obtaining liver biopsy (ultra sound guided).

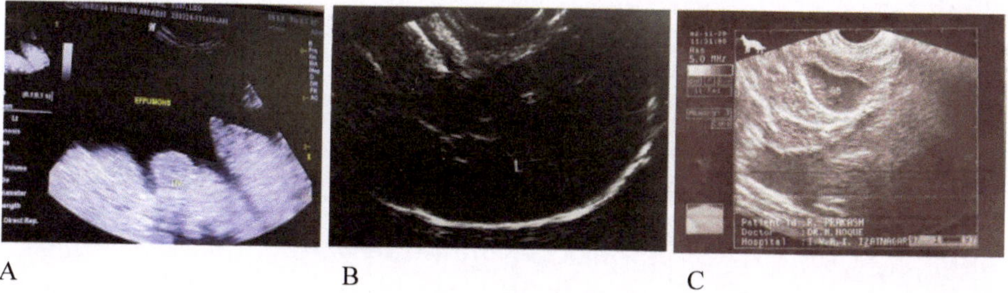

A B C

Figure 93: Ultrasonograms of the dogs showing cirrhotic liver with fluid **(A)**, hepatosis orhepatitis **(B)** and cholycystitis. **(C)** Computed Tomography (CT scan) and Magnetic Resonance Imaging (MRI)

CT scan and MRI are the advance imaging techniques being used in the diagnosis of hepatic parenchymal neoplasia in humans. These techniques are superior with improved accuracy as compared to abdominal ultrasound. Not much information is available on their performance in veterinary medicine. CT angiography is being used increasingly in canines for diagnosing congenital portosystemic shunts and other hepatic vascular diseases (Clifford *et al*.,2004).

(d) Nuclear Scintigraphy

This technique has been used to quantify liver function and to assess biliary tract patency in dogs. Transsplenic portal scintigraphy is recommended for the diagnosis of congenital PSS in dogs (Sura *et al*.,2007).

Biopsy

As sonography provides non-specific diagnosis of masses, nodules or effusion, tissue samples are necessary for histopathological examination for ascertaining the specific or definite diagnosis of liver diseases. Hepatic tissue samples can be obtained through ultrasound guided biopsy or exploratory laparotomy.

Urine Analysis

Urine analysis provides important data base. A decrease in urine specific gravity can be noted in dogs with portosystemic shunts or hepatic insufficiency. Bilirubinuria may be seen in normal dogs also. However, it is pathological in cats. Excessive bilirubinuria in dogs is suggestive of hemolytic or hepatobiliary disease.

Though, urate crystalluria (biurate -Figure94) has been reported in 40-70 % dogs with portosystemic shunts, it is not specific for hepatobiliary disease (Muller *et al*.,2000).

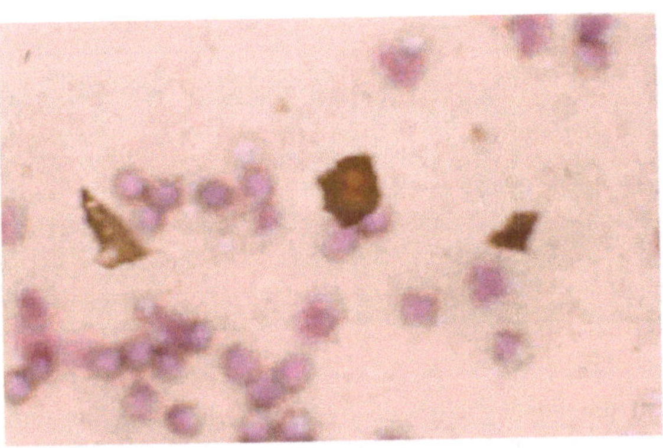

Figure 94: Biurate crystals in the urine of a dog diagnosed with intrahepatic portosystemic shunt.

Hemogram

Anemia and poikilocytosis may be recorded in dogs with chronic liver diseases. Target cells (Figure95) have been reported in chronic liver diseases. Microcytic anemia is common in dogs with portosystemic shunts. Hepatic neoplasm or disseminated intravascular coagulopathy may lead to the formation of schistocytes (Poldervaart *et al*., 2009). Changes in thrombocytes in hepatic disease are non-specific and inconsistent. Nevertheless, thrombocytopenia may be seen in cases with severe liver disease (Poldervaart *et al*.,2009). Thrombocytopenia is also observed in dogs with disseminated intravascular coagulopathy associated with liver disease or leptospirosis involving the liver. The hematological changes associated with liver diseases are also observed in many other diseases. Therefore, changes in hemogram are not of any specific diagnostic value except providing associated alterations to be taken care.

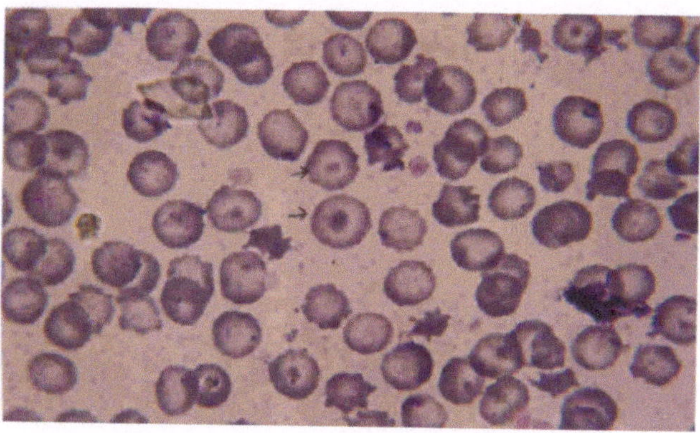

Figure 95: Blood smear of a dog is showing target cells.
The dog was later confirmed with intrahepatic portosystemic shunt.

References

Clifford, C.A., Pretorius, E.S., Weisse, C., Sorenmo, K.U., Drobatz, K.J., Siegelman, E.S. and Solomon, J.A. (2004). Magnetic resonance imaging of focal splenic and hepatic lesions in the dog. J. Vet. Intern. Med.18:330-338.

Dunayer, E.K. and Gwaltney-Brant,S.M. (2006). Acute hepatic failure and coagulopathy associated with xylitol ingestion in eight dogs. J. Am. Vet. Med. Assoc. 229: 1113-1117.

Gerritzen-Bruning, M.J., Ingh, T.S.G.A.M. and Rothuizen, J. (2006). Diagnostic value of fasting plasma ammonia and bile acid concentrations in the identification of portosystemic shunting in dogs. J. Vet. Intern. Med. 20: 13-19.

Kummeling,A., Teske, E. , Rothuizen, J. and Sluijs,F.J. (2006).Coagulation profiles in dogs with congenital portosystemic shunts before and after surgical attenuation. J .Vet .Intern. Med. 20:1319-1326.

Lakner, A.M., Bonkovsky, H.L. and Schrum, L.W. (2011). Micro RNAs:Fad or future of liver disease?. World J. Gastroenterol 17: 2536–2542.

Marolf, A.J. (2016). Computed Tomography and MRI of the hepatobiliary System and pancreas. Vet. Clinics North Am.: Small Anim. Practice 46: 481-497.

Muller,P.B., Taboada,J. and Hosgood, G.(2000). Effects of long-term phenobarbital treatment on the liver in dogs. J. Vet. Intern. Med.14, : 165-171.

Niles, J.D., Williams, J.M. and P. J. Cripps, P.J. (2001). Hemostatic profiles in 39 dogs with congenital portosystemic shunts. Vet. Surg, 30: 97-104.

Plourde, V., Gascon-Barre, M., Willems, B. and Michel Huet, P. (1988). Severe Cholestasis leads to vitamin D depletion without perturbing its C-25 hydroxylation in the dog. Hepatol. 8:1577-1585.

Poldervaart, J.H., Favier, R.P., Penning, L.C., Van Den, Ingh, T.S.G.A.M. and Rothuizen, J. (2009). Primary hepatitis in dogs. a retrospective review (2002–2006). J. Vet. Intern. Med, 23:.72-80.

Sura,P.A., Tobias,K.M., Morandi,F.,Daniel, G.B, and Echandi, R.L.(2007). Comparison of 99mTcO4– trans-splenic portal Scintigraphy with per-rectal portal scintigraphy for diagnosis of portosystemic shunts in Dogs. Vet. Surg. 36:654-660

Xenoulis, P.G. and Steiner, J.M. (2010). Lipid metabolism and hyperlipidemia in the dog. Vet. J. 183: 12–21.

12

Clinical Diagnostic Techniques in Nephrology and Urology

Nephrology

Nephritis and renal calculi are the two major problems leading to renal failure in canine and feline nephrology. Chronic renal failure may occur at any age but it is more common in geriatric dogs. Congenital renal diseases may also lead to renal failure at any age. Chronic renal disease or chronic renal failure is a progressive deteriorating condition as compensatory mechanism (glomerular hypertension and hyper filtration) further deteriorate the condition. Hence chronic renal disease remains lifelong. For quality life, an early diagnosis of renal failure is very important. The following techniques are used to diagnose chronic renal failure.

History

History of dogs with chronic renal failure is nonspecific. Anorexia, polydipsia, polyuria, weakness and loss in body weight are generally narrated by the owners. The disease is more common in geriatric dogs.

Clinical Manifestations

Generally clinical symptoms of chronic renal failure are in apparent or very mild .Isothenuria and azotemia do not develop until 65 to 70 % nephrons are dysfunctional or damaged. Polyuria, polydipsia, loss of weight, lethargy, vomiting and diarrhea are commonly seen in cases of chronic renal failure. Physical examination may show change in body condition score, dehydration, heart murmurs, hypertension, and anemia. Fundus examination may reveal vessel tortuosity and retinal detachment owing to systemic hypertension. Hematochezia or melena on rectal examination may be evident owing to gastrointestinal uremic ulcers.

Biochemical Indicators

Though serum creatinine and blood urea or blood urea nitrogen are important biomarkers of renal damage, their levels are also influenced by some external factors. Muscle wasting decreases creatinine level. BUN level increases in patients with gastric bleeding and on high protein diet; and decreases in dogs with mal nutrition or on protein restricted diet. Pre renal (decreased renal perfusion in dehydration, hypovolemia or hypotension) or post renal (ureteral obstruction) factors do increases azotemia (nitrogenous waste products blood urea, creatinine). Glomerular filtration rate is the gold standard test for renal function but not routinely used in clinical practice. Creatinine (mainly) and to lesser extent blood urea nitrogen are correlated with glomerular filtration.

Recently SDMA (serum symmetric dimethyl arginine) and CysC (cystatin C) has shown promise in detecting renal insult at an early stage. Of these CysC is the biomarker that can detect the earliest stage of CKD i.e. Stage 1 (Kim *et al*., 2020).

International Renal Interest Society (IRIS) has recommended staging of renal failure based on serum creatinine and or SDMA as stage 1 (Dogs creatinine < 1.4 mg/dl, SDMA < 18 µg/dl; Cats creatinine <1.6 mg/dl, SDMA <18.0 -µg/dl), stage 2 (Dogs creatinine < 1.4-2.8 mg/dl, SDMA < 18.0-35.0 µg/dl; Cats creatinine <1.6 – 2.8 mg/dl, SDMA <18.0- 25.0 µg/dl), stage 3 (Dogs creatinine < 2.9-5.0 mg/dl, SDMA < 36.0-54.0 µg/dl; Cats creatinine <2.9 – 5.0 mg/dl, SDMA <26.0-38.0 µg/dl), and stage 4 (Dogs creatinine >5.0 mg/dl, SDMA >54.0 µg/dl; Cats creatinine >5.0 mg/dl, SDMA >38.0 µg/dl).

Ultrasonography

It is a valuable tool in diagnosing and staging renal failure in dogs and cats. The most important ultrasonographic feature of chronic renal failure/chronic renal disease is diffuse increase in renal cortical hyper-echogenicity (Figure96), abnormal ratio of cortico-medullary junction and pyelectasia. These abnormalities increase significantly with the progression of IRIS stage (Perondi *et al.,* 2020). Detection of renal and urinary calculi is facilitated by ultrasonography.

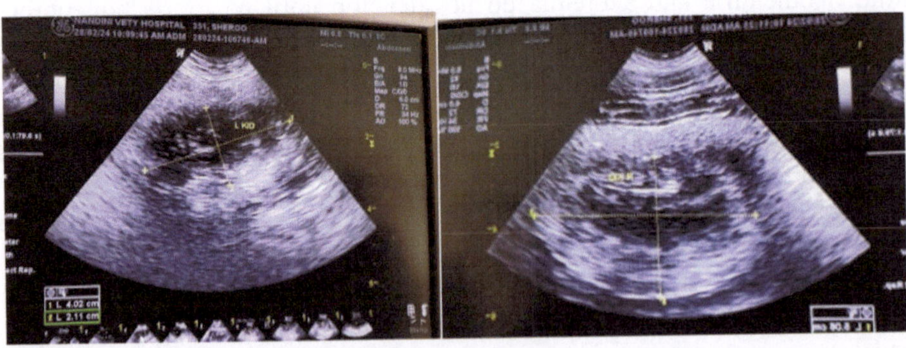

Figure 96: Ultrasonograms of dog showing diffuse increase in renal cortical hyper echogenicity of both kidneys suggesting chronic renal disease.

Ultrasonography can assist in differentiating acute and chronic renal disease. Chronic renal disease is characterized by small kidneys with irregular margins, hyper echoic cortices and poor corticomedullary differentiation. Whereas acute kidney disease is characterized by kidneys of normal or large size with normal architecture, hydronephrotic, and hyperechoic sonographic changes. Acute kidney disease is generally associated with perinephric fluid.

Radiography

It may be helpful in detecting stones or tumours.

Urine Analysis

Urine analysis is an important diagnostic technique that helps in diagnosing kidney and urinary tract diseases. Urine is subjected to routine examination including microscopy; and culture examination including antibiotic sensitivity. Routine urine analysis includes tests for specific gravity, pH, color, turbidity, glucose, ketone, bilirubin, blood and protein. Urine sediments are examined microscopically for pus cells, erythrocytes, crystals, other cells, casts and organisms. Urine in sterile container is used for culture examination and antibiotic sensitivity. For urine analysis fresh urine sample is preferable. If delay is expected, urine samples should be kept in refrigerator.

Normal urine is transparent and of yellowish or amber color. Its intensity depends on the volume of the urine produced and concentration of various products. Abnormal urine color may be caused by presence of endogenous or exogenous pigments. Red color of the urine (Figure 97) is due to the presence of RBCs in the urine. Coffee colored urine may be due to the presence of hemoglobin.

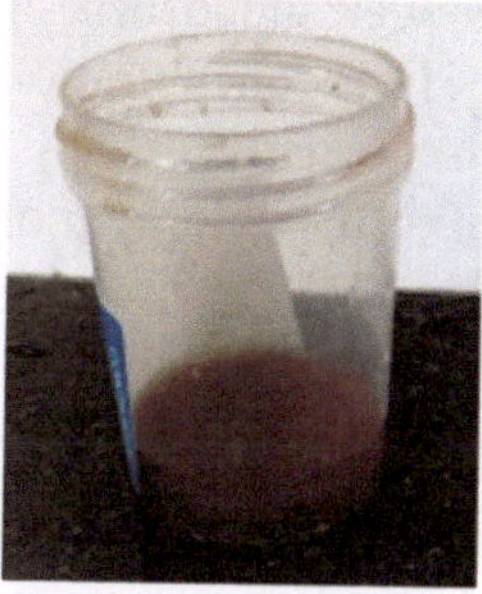

Figure 97: Showing red colored urine. Microscopic examination of the sample revealed the preponderance of RBCs.

Normal urine smells like ammonia. Bacterial infection may cause strong smell due to pyuria.

The urine specific gravity (SG) is highly variable depending on the fluid and electrolyte balance of the body. In healthy dogs it is 1.015. It increases in dogs with dehydration. Urine with low specific gravity in dehydrated or azotemia dogs may be due to renal failure, hypo- or hyperadrenocorticism, hyperkalemia, diabetes mellitus, hyperthyroidism. Specific gravity of the urine is also low in dog being treated with diuretic therapy. It also remains low (1.010) in dogs with diabetes insipidus. In diabetic dogs with glycosuria, specific gravity of the urine increases despite increased urine volume.

pH of the urine of healthy dogs is acidic and is influenced by diet , drugs and disease. Urinary infection with urease producing organism leads to alkaline urine pH.

No protein is detected in the urine of healthy dogs and cats. Proteinuria (presence of protein in the urine) can be due to pre-renal (fever, strenuous exercise, hyperthermia/heat stroke, hyperproteinemia or seizures), renal (nephritis) or post renal (inflammation, hemorrhage or infection) etiology. Whenever proteinuria is detected, it is to be interpreted along with the findings of specific gravity, urine pH and sediment microscopy. Alkaline urine may give false positive reaction and the presence of Bence –Jones protein may give false negative reaction.

Normally glucose is not present in the urine of healthy dogs and cats because renal threshold for glucose is around 180 mg/dl in dogs and 240 mg/dl in cats. With euglycemia, the amount of filtered glucose is less than the renal threshold, and all of the filtered glucose is reabsorbed in the proximal renal tubules. The presence of glucose in the urine (glycosuria) can be ascribed to hyperglycemia (owing to diabetes mellitus, excessive endogenous or exogenous glucocorticoids, or stress) or from a proximal renal tubular defect (primary renal glucosuria or Fanconi syndrome). Whenever glucosuria is detected, blood glucose level should also be monitored. High concentration of ascorbic acid or formaldehyde in urine may give false negative results. The contamination of urine sample with hydrogen peroxide, chlorine, or hypochlorite (bleach) may give false positive results.

Ketone bodies are not detected in the urine of healthy dogs. Routine test for ketone detects acetone and acetoacetic acid but not beta- hydroxybutyrate. The presence of ketone bodies in the urine (ketonuria) is suggestive of ketosis (secondary to diabetes mellitus in dogs), low carbohydrate diet in cats or prolonged fasting/starvation.

The presence of bilirubin in the urine (bilirubinuria) indicates that the amount of conjugated bilirubin has exceeded the renal threshold. It may occur in liver disease or hemolysis. A small amount of bilirubin in the concentrated urine may be normal. False positive result may be associated with pigmenturia. Urine containing large amount of ascorbic acid may yield false negative result.

Healthy dogs may normally have a small amount of urobilinogen (a product formed from bilirubin by intestinal microflora). Its level is increased in dogs with hyperbilirubinemia and it may absent in cases of biliary obstruction. Occult blood test detects intact erythrocytes, hemoglobin and myoglobin. A positive occult blood test indicates hematuria, hemoglobinuria or myoglobinuria.

For microscopic examination, the urine is centrifuged at 1,000–1,500 rpm for 3–5 min. The supernatant is decanted leaving a very small volume of urine (0.5 ml) and the sediment. The sediment is suspended in the small volume of the urine by tapping the tip of the conical tube against the table several times. A few drops of the sediment are transferred on to a glass slide and covered with a cover slip and examined under low (for crystals, casts and cells) and high power (for cells and bacteria) of the microscope. New methylene blue or modified Wright stain can be used to identify cells in air dried slides. Erythrocytes in unstained slides appear as small and round bodies having a slight orange tint and smooth appearance (Figure98). Number of erythrocytes in urine of healthy dogs remain < 5 per high power field. Increased number of erythrocytes in the urine is suggestive of hematuria. It may be due to urinary infection and or crystalluria. Urine collection by catheterization or cystocentesis may also cause hemorrhage. White cells in the urine are also termed as pus cell (Figure98). Their number in the urine of healthy dogs remains limited to 4-5 per high power field. Increase in white blood cells (leukocytes) per high power field in the urine is suggestive of urinary tract inflammation, infection, trauma or tumor. Transitional epithelial cells may be detected in urine as a contaminant or due to transitional call carcinoma. Squamous cells may be seen in cases with squamous cell carcinoma. Casts are elongated cylindrical structures. Hyaline casts, epithelial cellular casts, granular casts and waxy casts may be seen. Hyaline casts are seen in dogs with fever, exercise and renal disease. Epithelial cellular casts indicate renal tubular disease. Fatty casts are not common but may be seen with disorder of lipid metabolism. Few hyaline or granular casts are considered as normal but their large number is suggestive of renal disease. The presence of organisms in aseptically collected urine indicates infection. Small number of the organism may be due to contamination from lower urogenital tract. Organisms can be confirmed by staining as well as culture examination. Sometimes fungal hyphae, yeast and parasitic ova may be seen in the urine sediment. Crystals (Figure98) in the urine suggests crystalluria. Crystalluria and urolithiasis are not the same.

Uroliths may be without crystalluria. Crystals in the urine are influenced by the pH of the urine, urine temperature, concentration of the crystallogenic material and the time lapse between urine collection and examination. In dogs, urine crystals of struvite (Figure98), calcium oxalate (Figure98), urate, cysteine and bilirubin are commonly seen. Fat droplets (Figure98) in the dog's urine can be mistaken as erythrocytes. But these vary in size and tend to float on a different plane of focus. These droplets are not pathological. In the urine of male dogs detection of spermatozoa is a common finding.

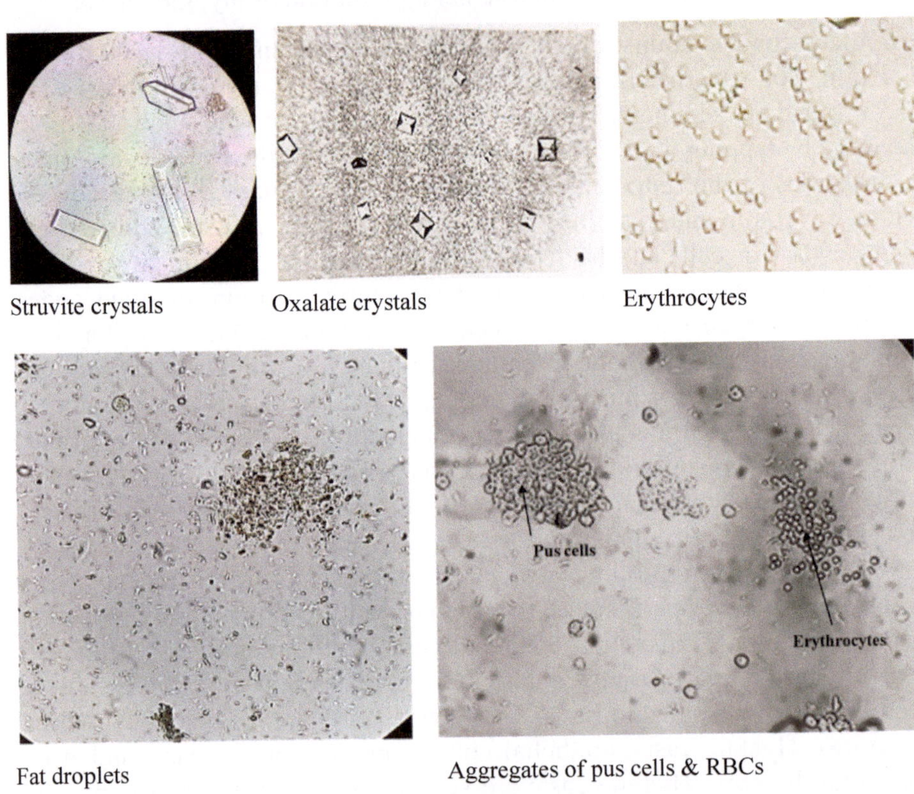

Figure 98: Microscopic examination of urine sediments showing struvite crystals, oxalate crystals, erythrocytes fat droplets and aggregates of pus cells and erythrocytes.

Urology

Urology is a branch of medicine related to diseases of lower urinary tract including prostates in male in human medicine. In veterinary medicine, urology is not dealt separately as a specialty but entire urinary system right from kidneys, ureters, urinary bladder, prostates to urethra is considered as one system. In humans, urinary bladder, urethra and prostate falls under lower urinary tract and their diseases are considered under the specialty of urology. With the same analogy, diseases of urinary bladder (cystitis, crystalluria, calculi in U.B., urinary bladder tumor), urethra (urethritis, stenosis due to calculi or neoplasm) and prostate (prostatitis, benign hyperplasia of prostate, prostatic abscess, prostatic neoplasm) in dogs may be considered under urology. But symptomology of diseases under urology and nephrology is overlapping and almost similar making it difficult to differentiate upper and lower urinary tract involvement. Diagnostic techniques described under nephrology are also employed for the diagnosis of the lower urinary tract diseases. Urine collection and blood tests are commonly the first steps in diagnosing and screening urologic conditions. Imaging techniques such as pyelogram, cystography, CT scan, ultrasound assists in the diagnosis of blockages, tumors and other abnormalities. Cytometry and urine flow tests are conducted in humans to monitor urinary function.

Diagnostic tests in urology begins with a simple physical examination and digital rectal exam (to evaluate prostate glands). The most common clinical signs related to diseases of urinary bladder, urethra and prostates (in males) in dogs are hematuria, stranguria, pollakiuria, urinary incontinence, or urinary scalding (Bartges, 2004). But none of these are specific to any particular disease and fail to differentiate urinary tract infection, urolithiasis, micturition disorders or prostate diseases. Application of blood test (creatinine, BUN, prostate specific antigen), urine analysis (routine, microscopic and culture) and imaging techniques (ultrasound, x-ray, pyelogram, cysto-urethrogram and cystoscopy) is in no way different than that described under nephrology for the diagnosis of renal diseases. Prostate specific antigen test is primarily used to screen for prostate cancer. Radiography can detect well-formed calculi (Figure99). Ultrasonography is of great advantage in the diagnosis of cystitis, bladder tumor, bladder calculi, crystalluria, hematuria, and prostate diseases (Figure100). Urine examination is imperative for detecting urinary tract infection, nature of crystalluria and occult hematuria.

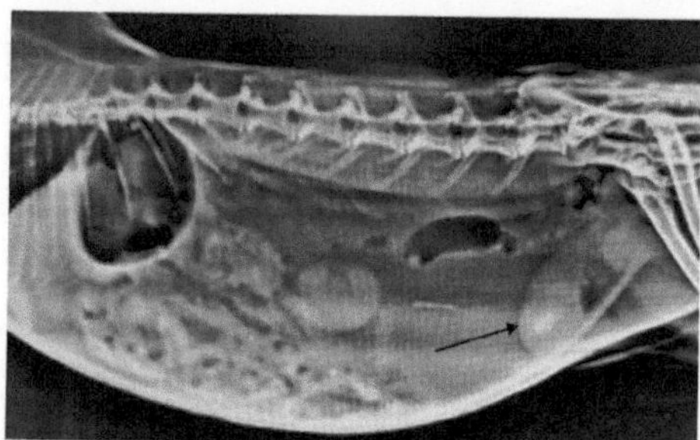

Figure 99: Radiograph showing calculi in the urinary bladder (marked with black arrow).

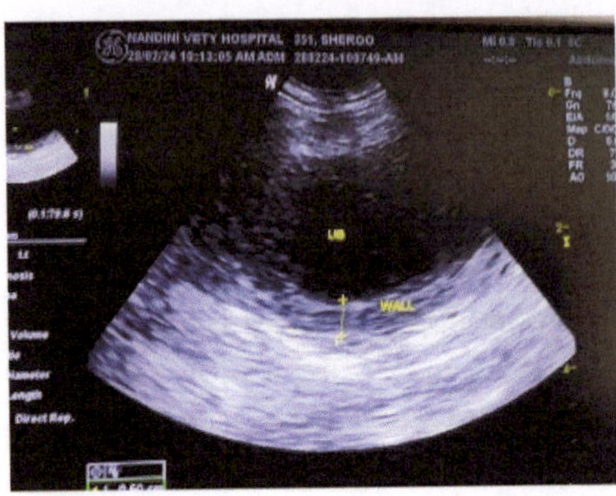

Cystitis

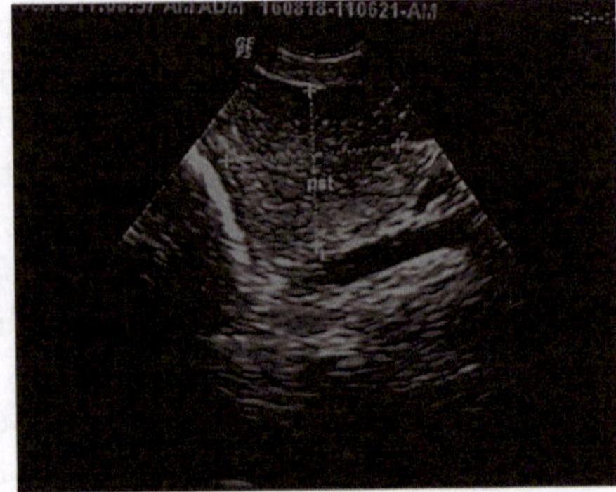

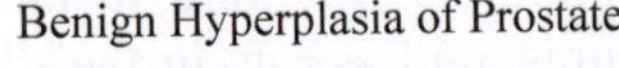

Benign Hyperplasia of Prostate

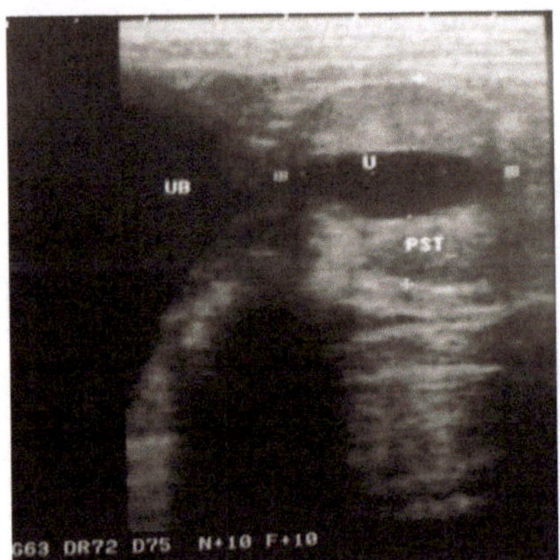

BHP pressing the urethra

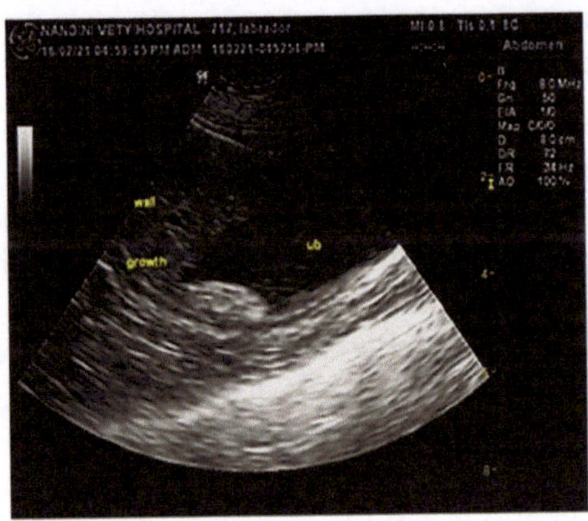

Tumor in Urinary Baldder

Figure 100: Ultrasonogram of dogs showing different diseases (cystitis, benign hyperplasia of prostate and urinary bladder tumor.

References

Bartges, J.W. (2004) . Diagnosis of urinary infections. Vet. Clin.-Small. Anim. 3:4923-4933.

Kim, J., Lee, Cang-Men. and Kim, Ha-Jung (2020). Biomarkers for chronic renal disease in dogs: comparison study. J.Vet.med.Sci. 82:1130-1137.

Perondi, F., Lipi, I., Marchetti,V.,Bruno,B., Borrelli, A., and Citi,S. (2020). How ultrasound can be useful for staging chronic renal disease in dogs: Ultrasound findings in 855 cases. Vet. Sci. 7(4):147. doi: 10.3390/vetsci7040147. PMID: 33019496; PMCID: PMC7712280.

13

Clinical Diagnostic Techniques in Neurology

Clinical diagnostic techniques in neurology are generally employed to confirm the existence of neurological disorder and also to localize the lesion.

Equipment/Instruments for Neurological Examination

- Reflex hammer.
- Cotton tip applicator.
- Pen torch light or transilluminator.
- Cotton balls.
- Haemostats.
- Lens.

Anesthesia/ Sedative

- Generally no anesthetic/ sedative is needed for neurological examination.

Place of Neurological Examination

- Neurological examination should preferably be conducted in a calm and quite room/place without any disturbance.
- For detecting subtle defects, non-slippery rough surface should be available.

Examination Procedure

Neurological examination is conducted to evaluate mentation, posture and gait, cranial nerves, spinal reflexes, postural reaction, palpation of spine and muscle, and assessing pain perception. All details are to be clearly noted.

(a) Evaluation of Mentation

It is a visual assessment of the patient (Figure101). Whether, the animal is normal (bright, alert, responsive, calm), dull or obtund (drowsy, inattentive but reactive to auditory stimuli such as calling its name, noise, clapping), stuporous (sleepy needing strong stimulation to show reaction), comatose (unconscious) or showing behavioral changes (agitation, aggression, dementia or obsessive compulsive behavior).

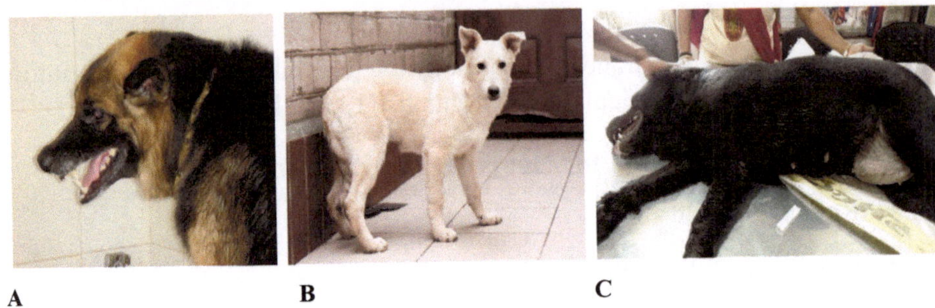

A **B** **C**

Figure 101: Dogs showing different mentation. **A.** An aggressive dog. **B.** An alert dog. **C.** A comatose dog

(b) Assessing posture

The orientation of the animal is to be noted. Whether the spine is normal, curved dorsally (kyphosis) or curved ventrally (lordosis). Whether the head is held normally or tilted. Neck and head is aligned normally or turned. The dog is assessed in standing position as standing normally (Figure102 A) or wide based stance. Upright position is the normal posture. Abnormality in posture is an indication of a lesion anywhere along ascending or descending pathways in the peripheral or central nervous system. Marked abnormalities in postural reactions without any change in gait is suggestive of a lesion in cerebral cortex. Head tilt (Figure102 B) is suggestive of disease affecting the vestibular system. Fore brain lesions may lead to head turn. Postures such as swaying, leaning on objects or wide based stance suggests cerebellar or vestibular system dysfunction.

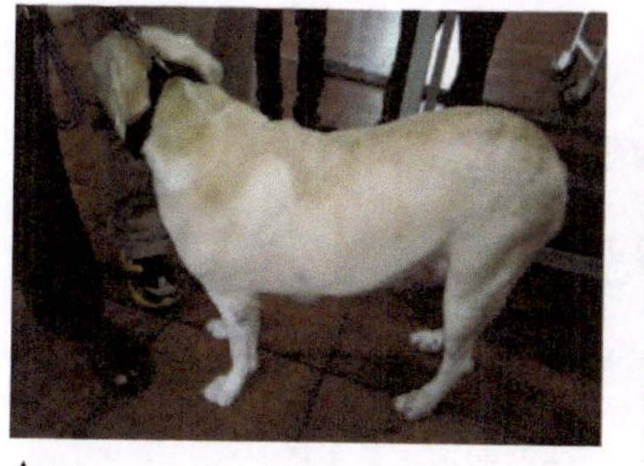

A

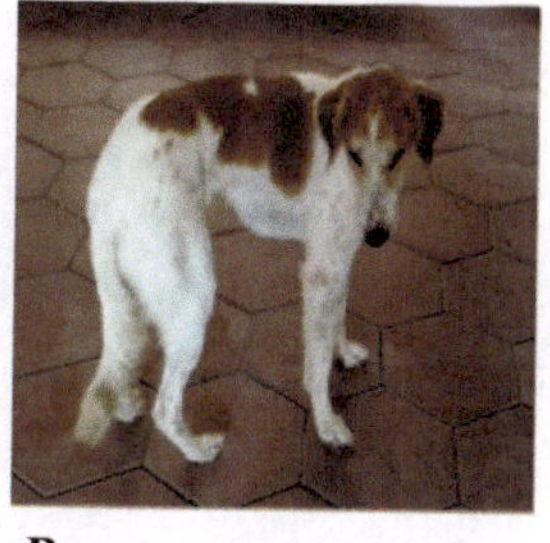

B

Figure 102: Different postures in dogs. **A.** Normal posture. **B.** Head tilt posture.

Postural reaction assessment - It is done by paw replacement, hopping, wheel barrowing, extensor postural thrust, and hemi walking.

Paw replacement test (Figure103) is conducted by flexing the paw with the help of few fingers (dorsum of the paw is on the non-slippery floor without bearing weight) and observing its return to normal position. The dog is supported under the chest (when the test is conducted for fore limbs) or pelvis/ caudal abdomen (when the test is done for the hind limbs), to prevent loss of balance at the time of paw flexion.

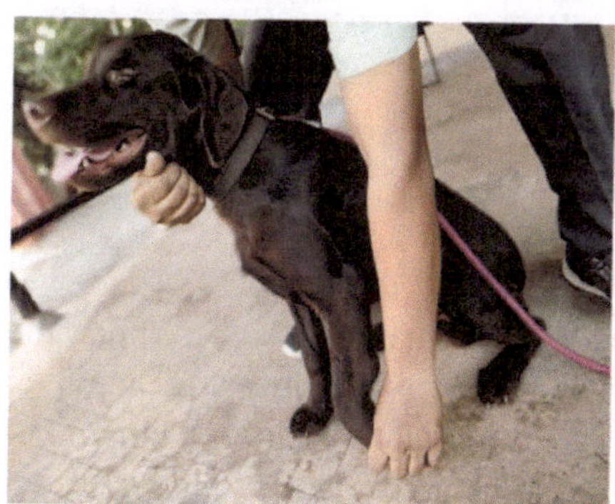

A

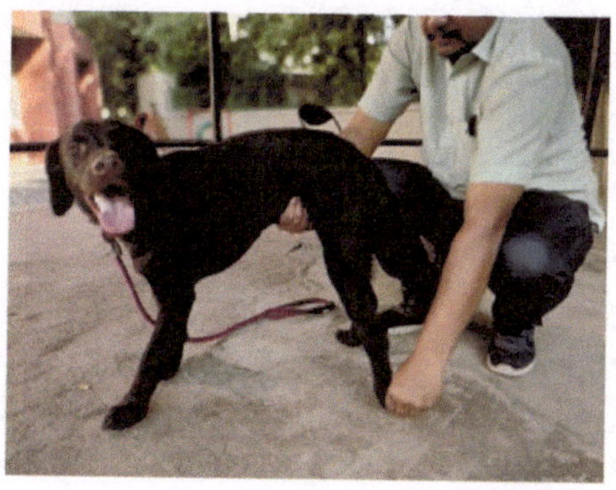

B

Figure 103: Paw replacement test in dogs. For paw replacement test in thoracic limb the dog is supported under the chest and the toe is flexed **(A)**. For paw replacement test in pelvic limb the dog is supported under the caudal abdomen or pelvis and then the toe is flexed **(B)**. Returning of paw to normal position is noticed.

Hopping test (Figure 104) is done by holding the patient in such a manner that all its weight is on one limb and the animal is moved forward or laterally. Normal animal hops on the limb. Each limb is tested individually.

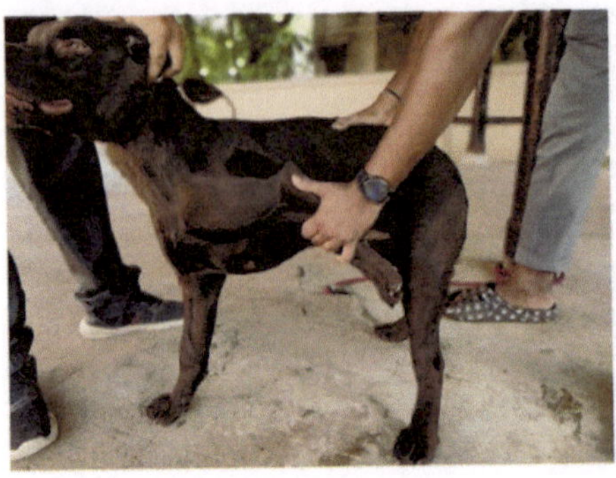
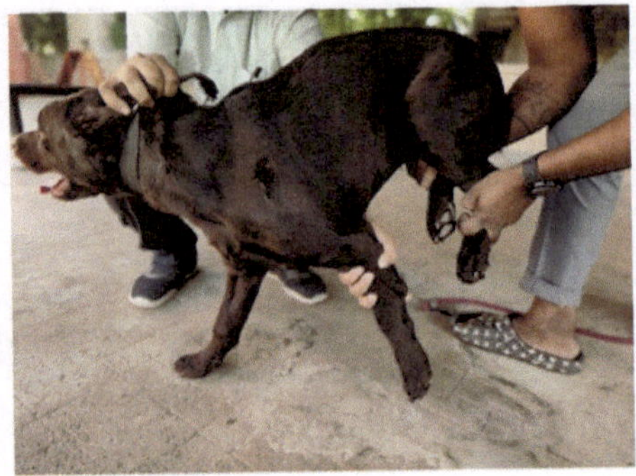

Figure 104: Hopping Test in dogs.

Wheel barrowing test (Figure 105) is conducted by supporting the dog under abdomen and lifting the hind limbs from the ground, allowing the animal to bear weight on its fore limbs (thoracic limbs) and then move the animal forward in the manner as wheel barrow is pushed. Normal dogs walk forward with coordinated movement.

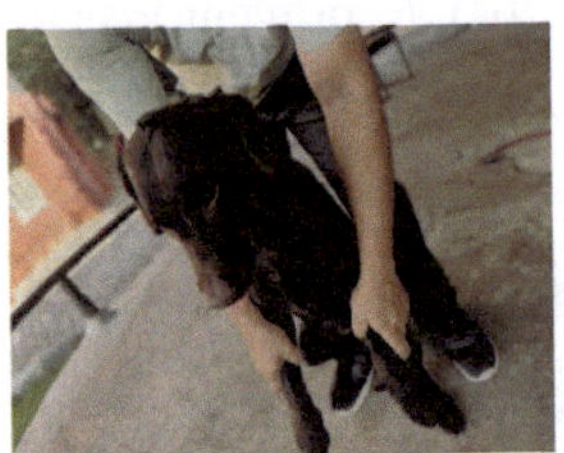
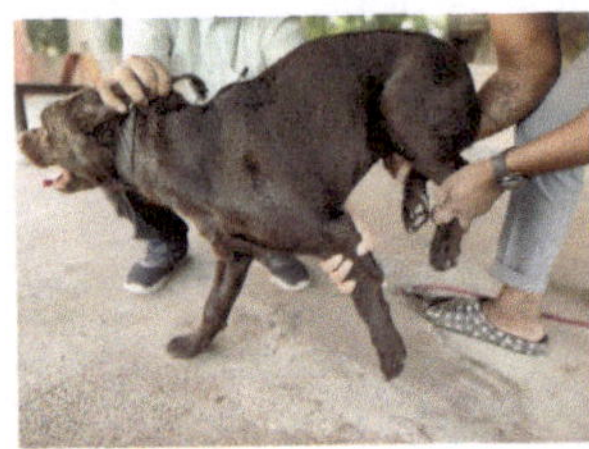
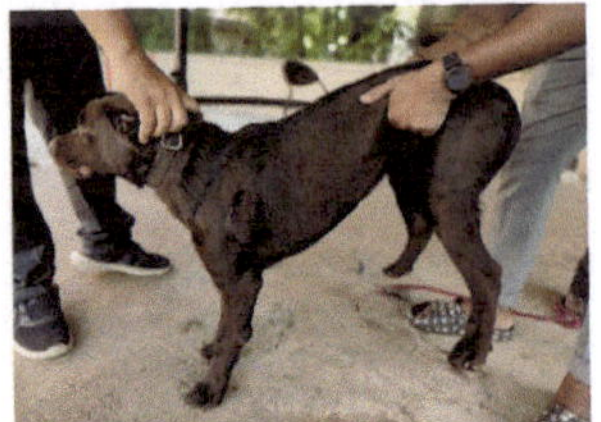

Figure 105: Wheel –barrow test in dogs

Extensor postural thrust test is conducted by supporting the dog under the thorax to lift fore limbs from the ground and allowing weight bearing on pelvic (hind) limbs .Then the animal is moved in symmetric walking movements to achieve a position of support. The dog should not be walked backwards (i.e., reverse wheel barrowing).

Hemi-walking test is conducted by lifting the front and rear limbs of one side and all weight bearing on the limbs of opposite side (if fore and hind limbs of left side are lifted then weight bearing is on the fore and hind limbs of right side). The dog is forced to hop with the limbs on the ground and the lateral walking movement is evaluated.

Postures such as ophisthotonus (dorso reflection of head and neck), decerebrate (all four limbs extended), decerebellate (extended thoracic limbs with flexed pelvic limbs) or Schiff-Sherrington (increased tone in thoracic limbs and hind limb paralysis) may be observed rarely.

(c) Assessment of the gait

Gait is to be observed from the front and back while the animal is walking in a straight line. For detecting subtle gait defects, the animal is to be observed while going up and down the stairs. Gait abnormalities are described as mix of weakness, ataxia, paresis/plagia or lameness. Ataxia (Figure106) is classified as proprioceptive (symmetric and mild incoordination), vestibular (asymmetric, falling or drifting to one side of mid line), or cerebellar (symmetric, bouncy gait with hypermetria without loss of strength in limbs). Paresis is characterized by reduced voluntary motor function. It is associated with certain degree of weakness. It may be neurogenic or muscular. While plegia (Figure107) is characterized by loss of motor function. It may be monoplegia (single limb paralysis), hemiplegia (one side body paralysis), paraplegia (hind limb paralysis) or tetraplegia (all four limbs paralysis). Lameness can be either of orthopedic or neurologic origin. Motor function should also be assessed. Tetraparetic/plegic dogs or cats require support under the pelvis. Animals are encouraged to move forward to see their voluntary movement. Motor function can be assessed by observing response on calling its name and walking with the animal. Response on touching is a reflex action and should not be considered voluntary movement.

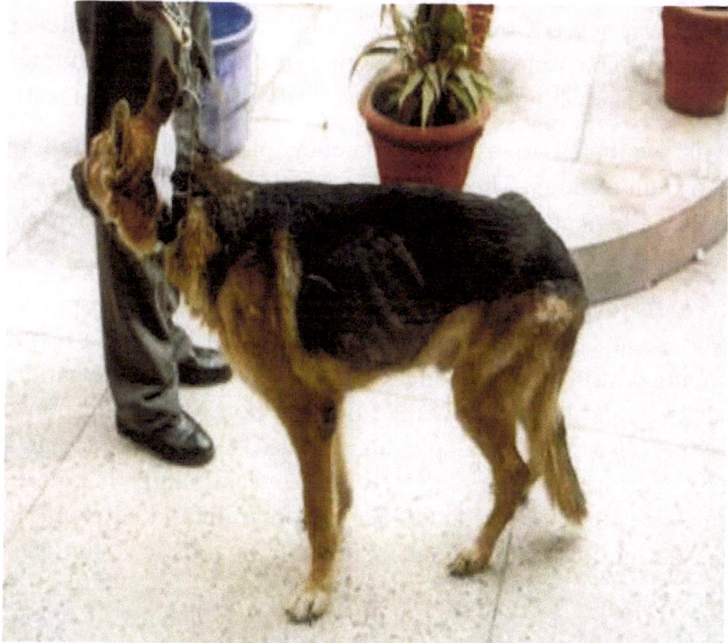

Figure 106: Hind limb ataxia in a German Shepherd

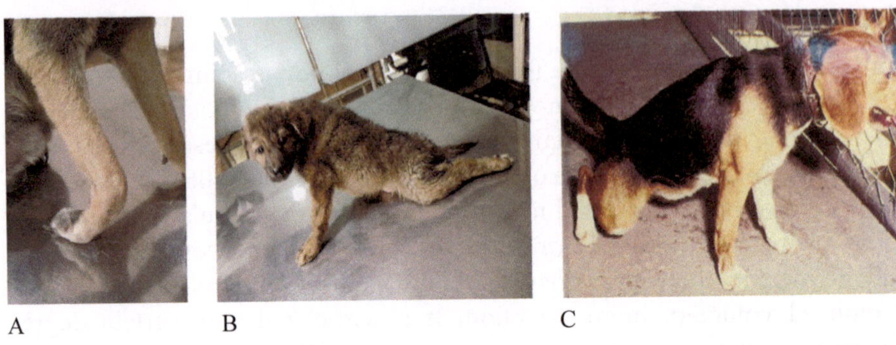

A B C

Figure 107: Plegia in dogs. **(A)** Right fore limb paralysis in a male German Shepherd.)Note the paw is flexed and the dog is not able to keep the paw in right position. **(B)** Paraplegia in a three month old non-descript dog caught by other dog. **(C)** Paraplegia in another dog. Note there is complete loss of motor function in the hind limbs.

(d) Cranial Nerve Evaluation

Cranial nerves are peripheral nerves originate from brainstem and perform both sensory and motor functions. There are 12 cranial nerves namely olfactory (CN I), optic (CN II), oculomotor (CN III), trochlear (CN IV), trigeminal (CN V), abducent (CN VI), facial (CN VII), vestibulocochlear (CN VIII), glossopharyngeal (CN IX), vagus (CN X), spinal accessory (CN XI) and hypoglossal (CN XII) nerve. Cranial nerves' evaluation is through reflexes (cranial nerve reflex and spinal reflex) and/or reactions (sensory pathway, motor pathway and cerebrum).Their function can be assessed through standard tests.

CN I (olfactory) is evaluated to ascertain patency of nares for smell in sniffers, detective or hunter dogs. The test is conducted by covering the eyes and presenting the food beneath the nose. The sniffing behavior is observed. Primary neurological problems related to CN I are rarely seen.

CN II (optic nerve) is evaluated by visual following, menace response, papillary light response and fundus examination. The visual following test is conducted by dropping cotton balls, moving a toy or ball in front of the patient and to see whether eyes and head follow the object or not. Menace response test (Figure108) is performed by waving a hand towards patient's face as a threatening gesture. Normally it is associated with eye blinking. It is used to assess the integrity of optic nerve, facial nerve, forebrain and cerebellum. Details of fundus examination are given in Chapter 14 Diagnostic Techniques in Ophthalmology.

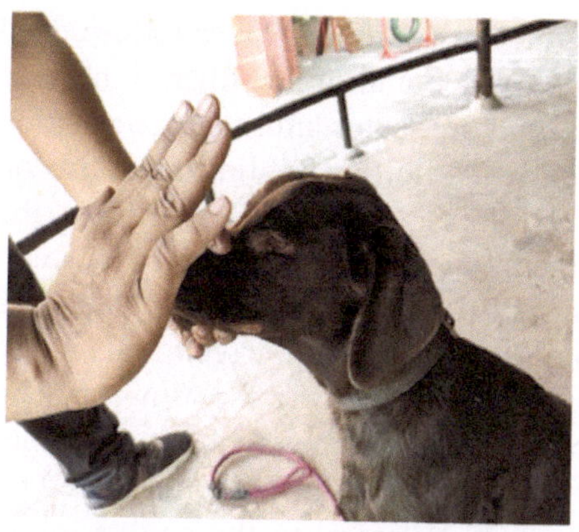

Figure 108: Performing a menace response test. The test is performed by waving a hand towards patient's face in a threatening manner. Normally it is associated with eye blinking.

CN III (Oculomotor) nerve's motor functioning is evaluated by pupil light response, eye position, and pupil size and observing for physiological nystagmus when turning the head. Pupillary light reflex test (Figure109) is done to assess the integrity of optic and oculomotor nerve. The test is done by shining a bright light into one eye and noting the constriction of pupil of the eye being tested as well as other eye also. CN III dysfunction causes ventrolateral strabismus, ptosis, mydriasis, unresponsive pupil, reduced or asymmetrical eyeball movement.

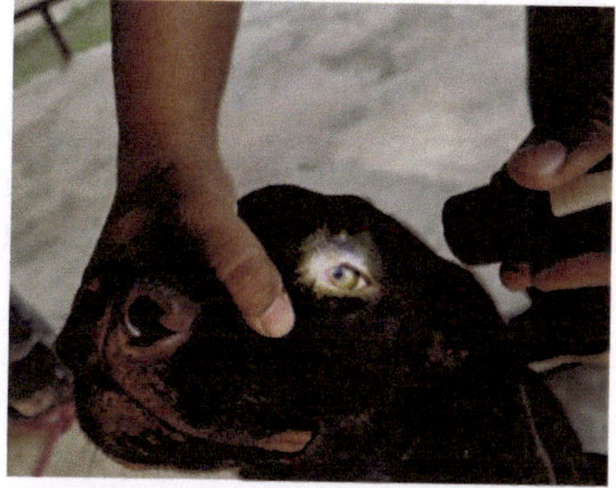

Figure 109: Performing a pupil light response test in a dog. The test is performed by shining a bright light into one eye and noting the constriction of pupil of the eye being tested as well as other eye also.

CN IV dysfunction leads to lateral deviation of the superficial retinal vein on ophthalmoscopic examination in the dog (round pupil). Motor functioning of CN IV nerve is evaluated by observing for dorsolateral rotation of the pupil and physiological nystagmus.

CN V (trigeminal) nerve has three branches (ophthalmic, maxillary and mandibular). Its sensory fibers innervate to face and motor fibers innervate to muscles of mastication (temporalis and masseter muscles). Sensation over all three branches should be examined. Eliciting a blink response on touching canthus of the eye (palpebral reflex – Figure110) indicates the integrity of the ophthalmic branch of trigeminal nerve. Wrinkling of face and a blink on touching or pinching the upper lip (Figure111) lateral to canine tooth indicates the integrity of the maxillary branch of trigeminal nerve. These responses also depends on the motor supply of the facial nerve. The patency of the maxillary branch is tested by pinching or touching the upper lip lateral to canine tooth. The patency of the mandibular branch is tested by pinching or touching the lower lip (Figure112) lateral to the canine tooth. Sensory testing of CN V nerve is done by evaluating nasal mucosa response, corneal reflex, palpebral reflex, trigeminofacial reflex (touching area of maxillary vibrissae and observing eye blink). Motor dysfunction of CN V nerve leads to atrophy of muscles of mastication (temporalis and masseter muscles – Figure113) leading to inability to close mouth. Palpebral reflex test is performed by touching medial and lateral canthi and observing the blink. Blink in response to touching medial and lateral canthi indicates intact palpebral reflex. This test is used to assess the integrity of trigeminal and facial nerves. Nasal stimulation response test is performed by touching the nasal mucosa on the medial aspect of each nare with a blunted probe (Figure114). Normally it elicits head withdrawal response. The test is used to assess the integrity of trigeminal nerve and the forebrain. In nut shell trigeminal nerve is evaluated by palpating masseter and temporal muscles for symmetry, atrophy, and pain; checking the jaw tone; looking for retraction response on touching the medial septum of the nose; observing for retraction response on touching globe; observing for blink response on touching medial canthus; and observing for snarl response on lip pinching

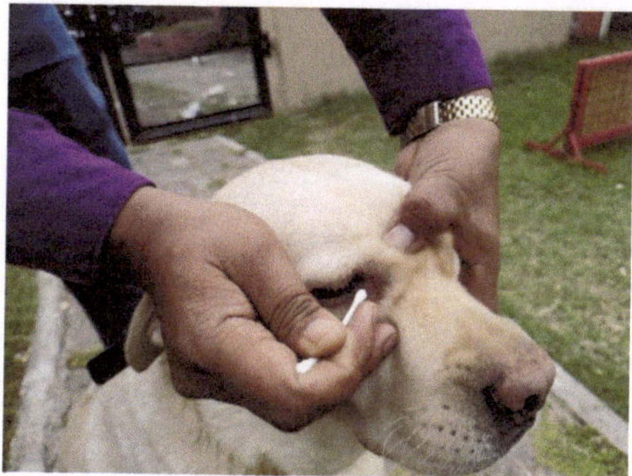

Figure 110: Testing of palpebral reflex in dog. The test is conducted by touching medial or lateral canthi and observing the blink response..

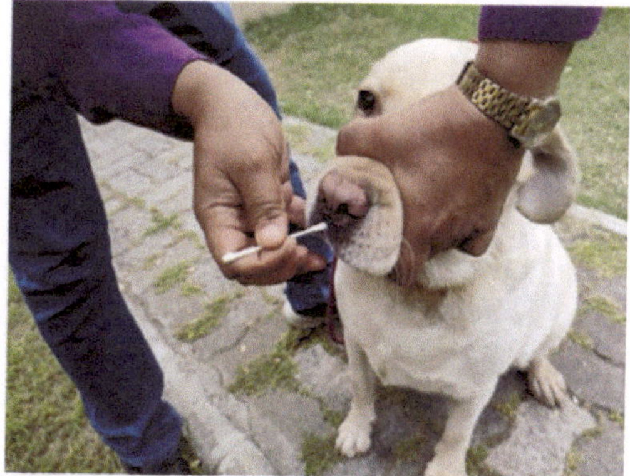

Figure 111: Testing of maxillary branch of trigeminal nerve. The test is conducted by touching or pinching the upper lip and observing wrinkling of face and a blink.

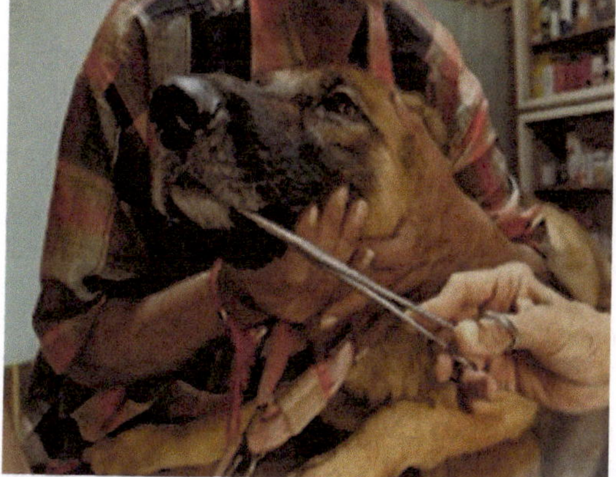

Figure 112: Testing of mandibulr branch of trigeminal nerve. The patency of the mandibular branch is tested by pinching or touching t

he lower lip lateral to the canine tooth

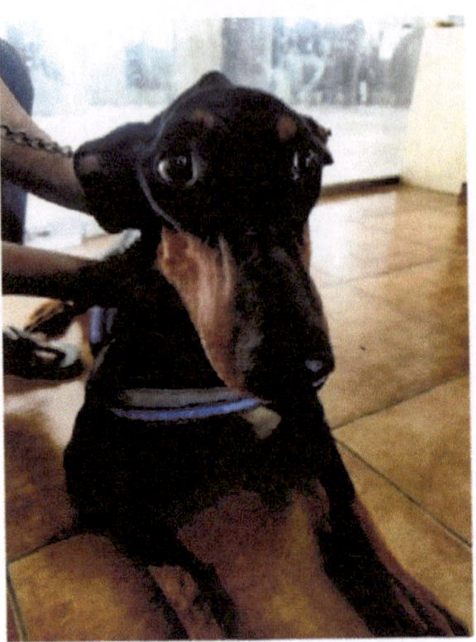

Figure 113: Dog showing atrophy of masseter and temporalis muscles

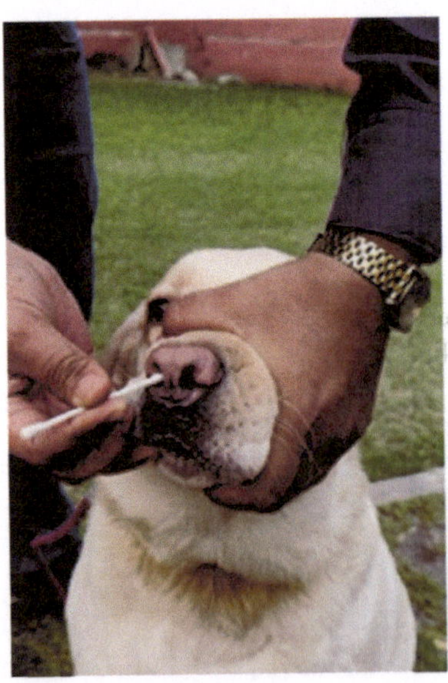

Figure 114: Nasal stimulation response test in dog. It is performed by touching the medial septum of the nose on each side with a cotton bud or blunted probe and observing head withdrawal response.

CN VI nerve (efferent) can be evaluated by corneal reflex (touching cornea and observing retraction – Figure 115), eye positioning, medial strabismus and physiological nystagmus. Dysfunction of CN VI leads to medial strabismus and reduced movement of eyeball.

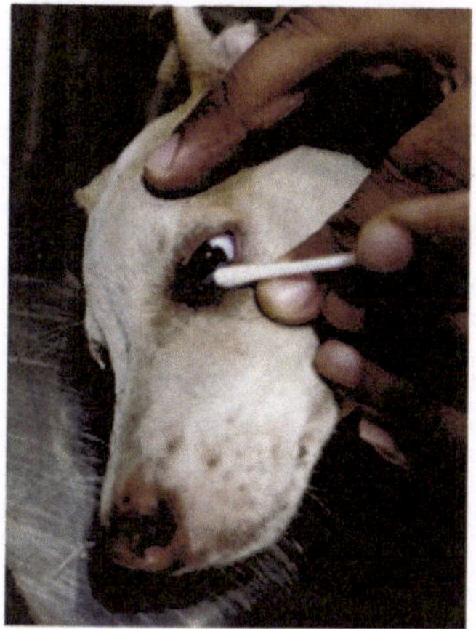

Figure 115: Testing of corneal reflex in dog. The test is performed by touching cornea with blunt object such as cotton buds and observing retraction

CN VII (facial) nerve innervates facial muscles, salivary and lacrimal glands. Its functioning is evaluated by menace response (detailed under CN II), palpebral reflex (detailed under CN V), corneal reflex (detailed under CN VI), Schirmer tear test (Figure 116A), ear flick response to medial pinna stimulation (Figure 116B) and observing for facial paralysis. Asymmetrical eyelid closure, a widened palpebral fissure, spontaneous blinking or drooping ears (Figure 116C) are suggestive of malfunctioning of the facial nerve.

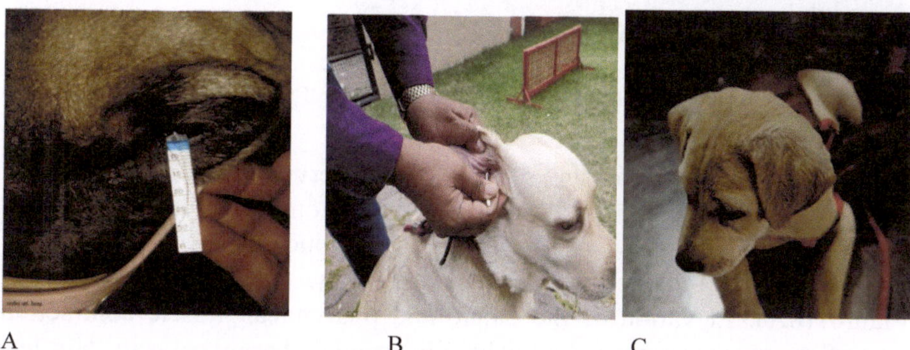

A B C

Figure 116: Showings tests for assessing facial nerve. **A.** Schirmer tear test for lacrimal gland functioning. **B.** Ear flick response to medial pinna stimulation. **C.** Drooping ear due to malfunctioning of facial nerve.

CN VIII (vestibulocochlear) nerve mediates hearing and vestibular function. Turning head toward loud unexpected noise is a normal response indicating the normal functioning of CN VIII nerve. Unilateral or partial deafness cannot be definitely ascertained by this crude test of response to unexpected noise.

The owner might observe signs of subtle hearing loss such as no readily response to calls. Head tilt (Figure117), nystagmus, ataxia, broad-based stance are suggestive of vestibular dysfunction. CN VIII nerve is evaluated by observing the head position and gait; and physiological nystagmus. Oculocephalic reflex test is performed by turning the head of the animal from side to side and observing the rapid movement of the eye in the direction of the head turned. The test is indicated to assess the integrity of the vestibulocochlear, oculomotor, trochlear, and abducent nerves.

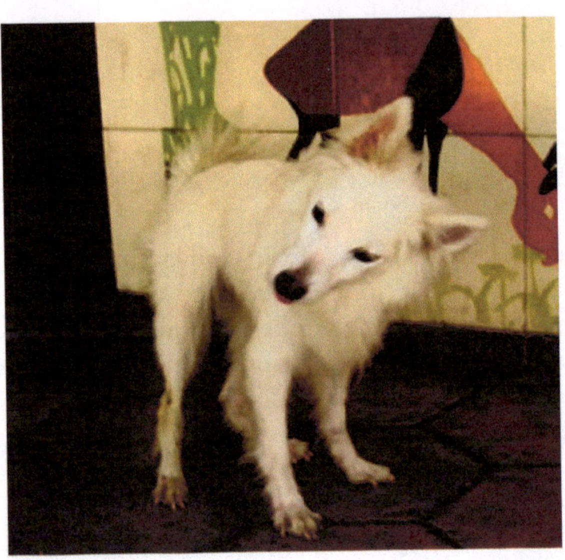

Figure 117: Pomeranian dog showing head tilt, an indication of vestibular dysfunction (CN VIII).

CN IX (glossopharyngeal) and CN X (vagus) nerves innervate (motor and sensory fibers) to the pharynx. Vagus nerve also controls laryngeal function. The functioning of these nerves is tested by touching (with the help of applicator stick) both left and right sides of the caudal pharyngeal wall (Figure118A). Elevation of the palate and pharyngeal muscle contraction (gag reflex) are the response to touching the caudal pharyngeal wall. This test is known as Gag reflex test. It is difficult to perform this test in temperamental dogs. Asymmetrical response is indicative of dysfunction. Functioning of CN IX and X nerves is evaluated by gag swallow reflex, observing any voice change or abnormal respiratory sound; and signs of coughing/ aspiration when eating or drinking. Vagus nerve can also be examined by observing laryngeal paralysis and assessing for mega esophagus and regurgitation by x-ray examination (Figure 118B).

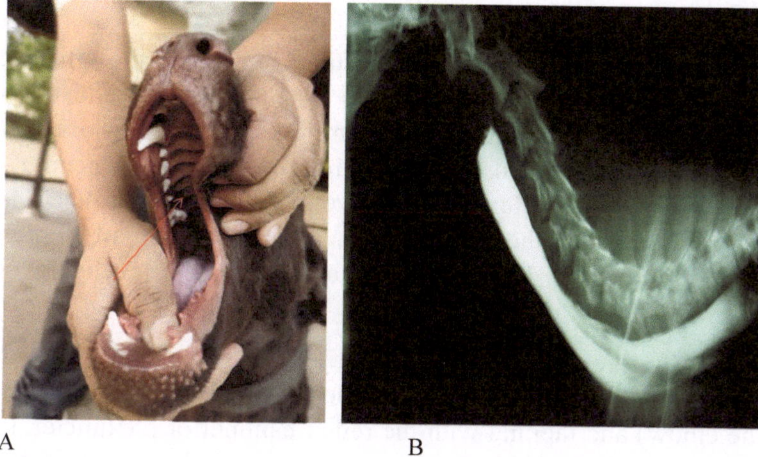

A B

Figure118: Tests for the functioning of glossopharyngeal and vagus nerves. **A.** Showing place for touching pharyngeal wall. Its stimulation results in gag reflex. **B.** Barium meal x-ray showing mega esophagus, an indication of malfunctioning of vagus nerve.

CN XI (spinal accessory) nerve (motor fibers) innervates to trapezius muscle. Atrophy of trapezius muscle is suggestive of CN XI abnormality. Functioning of CN XI nerve is evaluated by examining trapezius muscle and signs of left and right muscle asymmetry.

CN XII (hypoglossal) nerve innervate tongue muscles. Asymmetry, atrophy or deviation of tongue from normal position (Figure119) is indicative of hypoglossal nerve affection. Tongue function can be assessed by watching the dog drinking water. Changes in the symmetry of the tongue musculature and its voluntary movement are suggestive of nerve dysfunctioning.

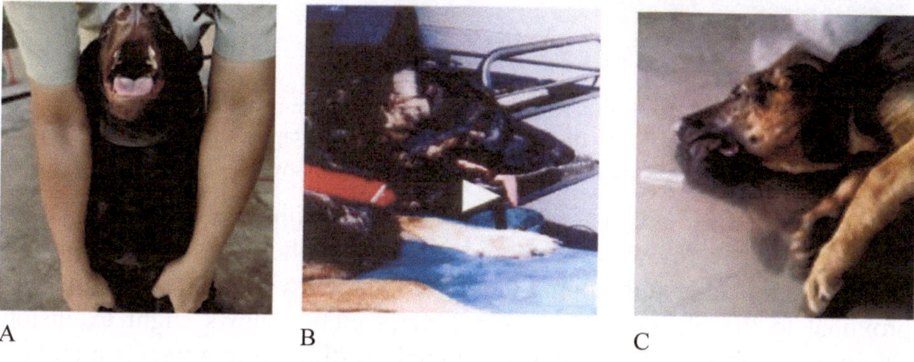

A B C

Figure 119: Dogs showing normal and abnormal functioning of hypoglossal nerve. Normal positioning of tongue indicative of normal functioning of hypoglossal nerve **(A)**. Tongue is hanging to its right side **(B)**.Tonge is hanging to its left side ©. Tonge postioning and asymmetry in Fig **B** and **C** is suggestive of dysfunctioning of hypoglossal nerve (CN XII).

(e) Spinal Reflexes

The integrity of sensory and motor components of the reflex arc and the influence of descending motor pathways on the reflex is tested by spinal reflexes. A reduction or absence of reflex is suggestive of complete or partial loss of either the sensory or motor nerves responsible for the reflex (lower motor neuron – LMN). While an exaggerated reflex is suggestive of a deformity or defect in the descending pathways from the brain and spinal cord that normally inhibit the reflex (upper motor neuron -UMN). Fore limb reflexes are less reliable for localizing lesions.

The Biceps reflex (Figure 120) is performed by pulling the thoracic limb slightly caudally, placing the index finger on the biceps tendon (cranial and proximal to the elbow) and tapping with the reflex hammer or pleximeter. In normal cases the elbow shows slight flexion. An absence or decrease in reflex is suggestive of a lesion involving spinal cord segments from C6 to T2 (LMN). While an exaggerated reflex is suggestive of a lesion cranial to spinal cord segment C6 (UMN).

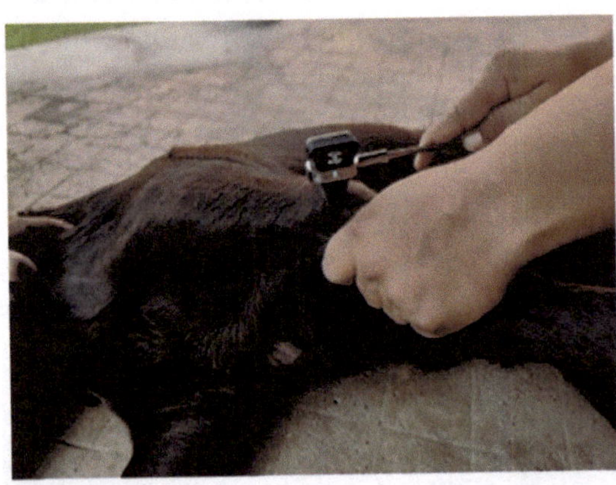

Figure 120: Performing a biceps reflex test in a dog. The thoracic limb (fore limb) is pulled slightly caudal placing an index finger on biceps tendon and tapping it with reflex hammer. Normal biceps reflex is associated with slight flexion of the elbow.

The triceps reflex (Figure 121) is performed with the animal in lateral recumbency. The elbow is flexed and abducted by holding the thoracic limb over the radius ulna and tapping the triceps tendon with a reflex hammer just proximal to the olecranon. In normal cases elbow shows slight extension. Eliciting of triceps reflex in normal animals is difficult to appreciate making the interpretation of lowered or absent triceps reflex a more difficult task. While an exaggerated reflex is suggestive of a lesion cranial to C7 (UMN).

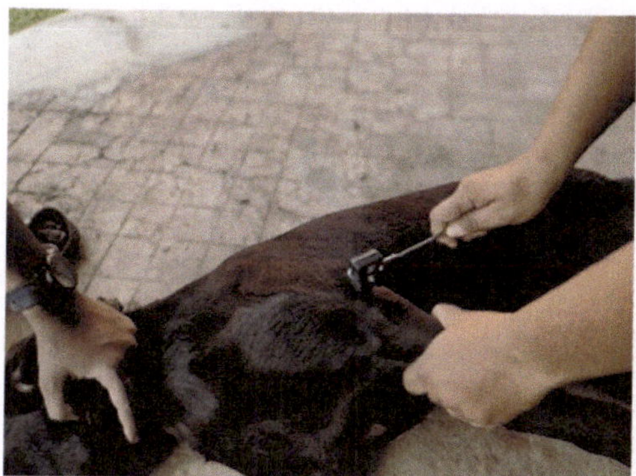

Figure 121: Performing a triceps reflex test in a dog. The elbow is flexed and abducted by holding the thoracic limb over radius –ulna and tapping triceps tendon with reflex hammer just proximal to olecranon. A normal reflex is associated with slight extension of the elbow.

The Patella reflex is a reliable test. It is performed with the animal in lateral recumbency supporting the uppermost pelvic (hind) limb by holding the hock with slightly flexed stifle and tapping the patellar ligament briskly with a reflex hammer (Figure 122). A single quick extension of the stifle is a normal response. An absence or reduced patellar reflex with flaccidity is suggestive of a lesion of sensory or motor component of the reflex arc (LMN). Loss of patellar reflex in one limb is suggestive of femoral nerve lesion. While loss of patellar reflex in both hind limbs indicates segmental spinal cord lesion (L4-L6). Hyper patellar reflex (exaggerated patellar reflex) with spasticity (increased muscle tone) along with signs of UMN dysfunction is suggestive of lesion in the spinal cord cranial to L4 segment (UMN). Exaggerated patellar reflex is also seen in loss of sciatic nerve integrity.

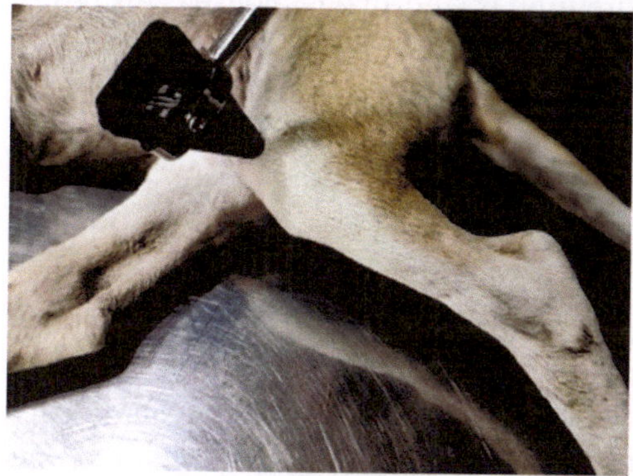

Figure 122: Performing a patellar reflex test in a dog. The uppermost pelvic limb is supported by holding the hock with slightly flexed stifle and briskly tapping the patellar ligament with reflex hammer. A single quick extension of the stifle is a normal response.

The gastrocnemius reflex is mediated via the tibial branch of the sciatic nerve and cord segment L5 to L7 and S1. This reflex is tested with the dog in lateral recumbency supporting the uppermost pelvic limb (hind leg) by placing a hand under the metatarsal bones with slightly flexed hock and striking gastrocnemius tendon briskly with a reflex hammer (Figure 123). Extension of the hock followed by flexion is a normal reflex.

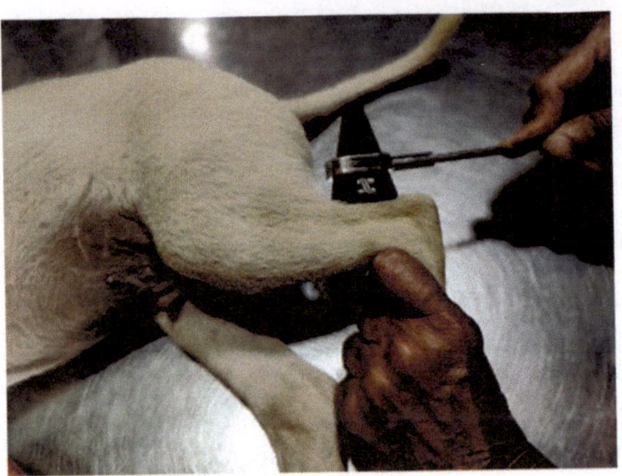

Figure 123: Performing gastrocnemius reflex test in a dog. The reflex is tested with the dog in lateral recumbency supporting the uppermost pelvic limb by placing a hand under the metatarsal bones with slightly flexed hock and striking gastrocnemius tendon briskly with a reflex hammer. Extension of the hock followed by flexion is a normal reflex.

The withdrawal reflex (Figure 124) should be tested in both fore and hind limbs. The dog is placed in lateral recumbency for testing the withdrawal reflex in fore (thoracic) limbs. On application of the least harmful stimulus (pinches) to the foot, flexion of the entire limb is a normal response. This reflex is primarily mediated through spinal cord segments C6-T2. Any abnormality in withdrawal reflex (absence or depression) indicates a lesion of spinal cord segments (C6 to T2) or of the peripheral nerves (LMN). Exaggerated withdrawal reflexes associated with other signs of upper motor neuron (UMN) dysfunction are suggestive of a lesion cranial to spinal cord segment C6 (UMN). The withdrawal reflex in the pelvic limbs is tested in the similar manner described for thoracic limbs. Flexion of entire hind limb in response to stimulus is a normal response. The withdrawal reflex in pelvic (hind) limbs is mediated through spinal cord segments L6 to S1 and the sciatic nerve. Any abnormality in withdrawal reflex (absence or depression) indicates a lesion of spinal cord segments (L6 to S1) or of the peripheral nerves (LMN).If the withdrawal reflex is absent in only one limb, it is most likely due to a sciatic nerve lesion. Exaggerated withdrawal reflexes are suggestive of a lesion cranial to spinal cord segment L6 (UMN).

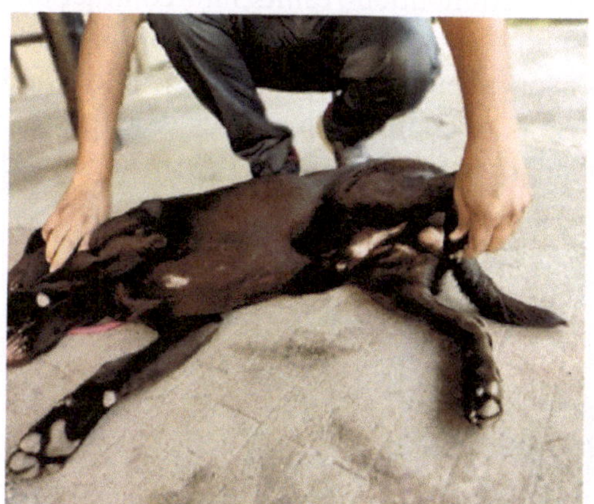

Figure 124: Performing a withdrawal reflex test in a dog. The dog is placed in lateral recumbency and a mild stimulus is applied to the foot web (pinching). Flexion of the entire limb is normal response. The test should be conducted in both fore and hind limbs.

The cutaneous trunci reflex is tested by applying pin-prick stimulus to the skin over the back starting from the lumbosacral region and continuing cranially (Figure 125). Twitching of the cutaneous trunci muscle on both sides of the dorsal midline, at the point of stimulation and cranially is the normal response to the pin-prick stimuli. Consistent absence of a response occurring only on one side (avulsion side) one or two segments caudal to the spinal cord lesion may be due to brachial plexus avulsion injuries.

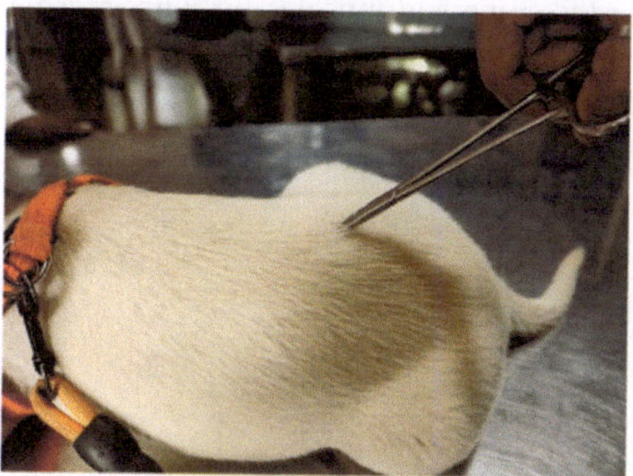

Figure 125: Performing a cutaneous trunci reflex test in a dog. The test is performed by applying pin prick stimulus to the skin over the back starting from the lumbosacral region and continuing cranially. Twitching of the cutaneous trunci muscle on both sides of the dorsal midline, at the point of stimulation and cranially is the normal response to the pin-prick stimuli.

The anal sphincter reflex is tested by gentle perineal stimulation with blunt forceps (Figure 126). Normally perineal stimulation results into contractions of the anal sphincter muscle. Anal sphincter reflex is mediated through the pudendal nerve (perineal nerve is sensory; caudal rectal nerve is motor) and spinal cord segments S1-S3. Absence or poor contraction of anus is suggestive of a lesion of sacral spinal cord or pudendal nerve lesion (LMN). An exaggerated response is suggestive of a lesion above the S1 spinal cord segment.

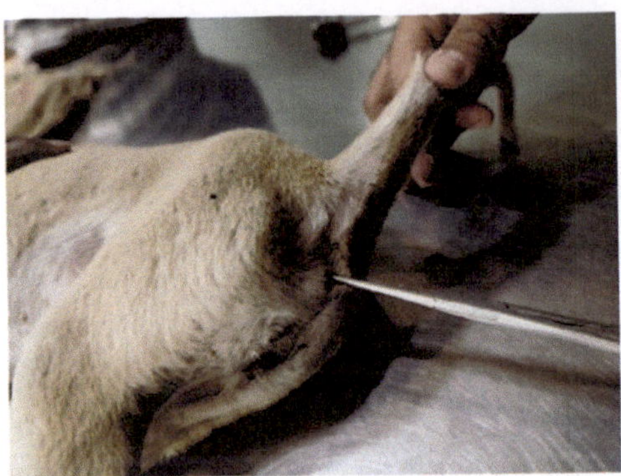

Figure 126: Performing an anal sphincter reflex test in a dog. The test can be conducted in standing or recumbent positions. A gentle stimulation with blunt forceps is applied in peineal region. It elicits contraction of the anal sphincter muscle is healthy dogs indicating an intact anal sphincter reflex

(f). Palpation

Palpation (Figure 127) is done along the spine and muscles for pain, muscle tone and atrophy. Neck is moved in all directions to check for pain. Dog undergone surgery or suffering from atlantoaxial subluxation or suspected fracture is not subjected to neck rotation.

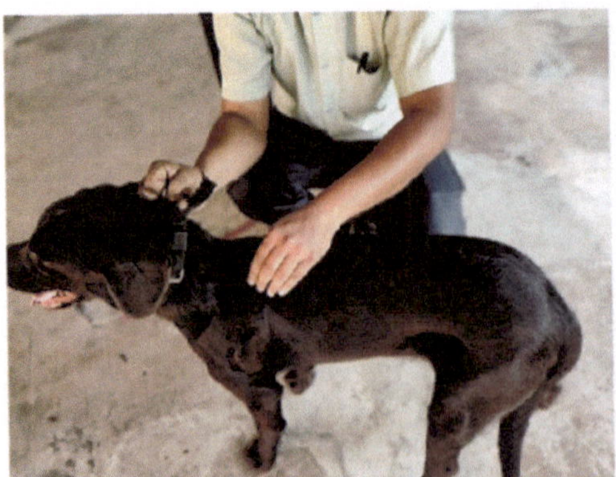

Figure 127: Performing palpation test in a dog. Palpation is conducted along the spine and muscles to observe pain, atrophy and muscle tone.

(g). Pain Perception

Pain perception is assessed in dogs with loss of motor function and young ones with signs of a sensory neuropathy. A conscious response (vocalizing, trying to bite, turning the head, whining, dilating pupils, increased respiratory rate) to pinching the toe web (using a hemostat) is suggestive of pain. Lack of deep pain perception carries a guarded to poor prognosis.

Cerebrospinal Tapping

Cerebrospinal fluid is an ultra-filtrate of the plasma produced by choroid plexus within the ventricular system and found in subarachnoid space surrounding the brain and spinal cord. The fluid is clear, colorless and transparent with few cells and protein. It plays an important role in providing physical support; pressure modulation; transport of metabolites, nutrients, and neurotransmitters; and maintenance of ionic balance (Di Terlizzi and Platt, 2009). Evaluation of cerebrospinal fluid is of diagnostic value in dogs and cats with central nervous system signs. As compared to blood, cerebrospinal fluid analysis provides more accurate reflection of ongoing pathology in brain, meninges and spinal cord.

Indications

Cerebrospinal fluid tapping is indicated in dogs and cats with seizures, incoordination, circling, nervous signs, and pain in neck or back, CNS disorders, encephalopathy and myelopathy. The animal suspected with an infectious or inflammatory disease, tumor, degenerative disease of the brain and or the spinal cord, are good candidate for examination of cerebrospinal fluid.

Contraindications

- Increased intracranial pressure as seen in space occupying lesion, cerebral trauma, hydrocephalus, and inflammatory diseases of central nervous system.
- Underlying coagulopathy.
- Atlanto-axial subluxation.
- Cervical trauma.

Risk Factors

- Anesthesia risk.
- Trauma to brain stem or spinal cord from the spinal needle.

- Invasion of infection if aseptic procedures are not maintained.

Material Needed

- Spinal needle (7- 9 cm, 22-20 gauge).
- Cotton swab.
- B.P. blade with handle.
- Sterilized test tubes, test tube with EDTA, and plain test tubes.
- Sterilized test tubes, test tube with EDTA, plain tubes
- Razor
- Rectified spirit
- Sterile surgical gloves

Sites for CSF Tapping

Cerebrospinal fluid can be collected from cistern magna (atlanto-occipital or cerebellomedullary cistern puncture) or lumbar puncture. In dogs and cats cistern magna site is preferred.

Preparation of the Site

The site for CSF tapping is prepared aseptically by shaving, cleaning and applying antiseptic on the skin.

Restrain and Control

Spinal tapping at cistern magna site is generally recommended under general anesthesia to reduce the risk of animal movement. Short acting barbiturate provides satisfactory anesthesia for dogs. For spinal tapping at lumbar site in large animals local anesthesia (xylocaine 2 %) may be used.

Positioning

The dog is placed in lateral recumbency with head and cervical vertebrae at the edge of the table. Skull is flexed to create a 90^0 angle with the cervical spine. The nose is slightly elevated to keep the long axis of the muzzle parallel to the table.

Tapping Procedure

Tapping procedure is done at the aseptically prepared site. For cisternal tapping (CMC tapping), a spinal needle with stylette (keeping it perpendicular to dorsal laminae of vertebral column) is inserted slowly at the level of atlanto-occipital space (mid line between occipital crest and the cranial edge of the wings of the atlas) in to the spinal column penetrating the duramater and arachnoid membranes to subarachnoid space. No resistance is felt as soon as the needle enters the subarachnoid space. Stylette is removed. A sterile syringe is attached to the spinal needle to draw out CSF or fluid can also be allowed to drip directly into the collection tube. Once CSF collection is completed, the needle is gently removed.

Lumbar tapping is comparatively more difficult to perform and is associated with more chances of blood contamination. Tapping at lumbar site is done in lateral recumbency with the pelvic limbs fully flexed. The appropriate intervertebral space is L5-L6 in dogs and L6-L7 in cats (Oliver and Lorenz, 1997). The needle (20 G) is inserted caudal to L6 perpendicular to the dorsal laminae of the vertebrae, along the cranial border of the caudal dorsal spinous process until it touches the bone of ventral aspect of the spinal canal. Insertion of the needle in the canal may cause a slight twitch of the tail or leg. The stylette is taken out and the fluid is collected. The flow of the fluid is slow and quantity of the fluid, that can be retrieved, is also less as compared to cisternal tapping.

Fluid Collection

CSF can be collected in EDTA tubes or plain sterile tubes. CSF collected in EDTA tubes is used for hematological evaluation. The volume of CSF collection should not be more than 1.0 ml/5 kg body weight in dogs and cats (Carmichael, 1998).

CSF Analysis

CSF should be processed for examination within 30-60 minutes of collection. It is subjected to physical, chemical, cytological and microbial examinations. Physical examination includes color, turbidity and coagulation. Indices of chemical examination are proteins, glucose, chloride, sodium, cholesterol, enzymes (lactic dehydrogenase, ALT and AST). Cytological examination of CSF includes total nucleated cells and differential cell count. CSF samples having high cell count and increased protein should also be subjected to cultural examination for isolation and identification of the organisms. Normal CSF contains total white cell up to 5 cells/µL and total protein as 10-25 mg/dl (much lower than blood).

References

Carmichael, N. (1998). Nervous system. In: Manual of Small Animal Clinical Pathology.

Davidson, M., Else, R. and Lumsden, J. (Eds.). British Small Anim. Vet. Assoc. Cheltenham, UK, pp. 235–240.

Di Terlizzi, R. and Platt, S.R. (2009). The function, composition and analysis of cerebrospinal fluid in companion animals: Part II – Analysis. Vet J. 180: 15-32.

Oliver, J.E. and Lorenz, M.D. (1997). In: Handbook of Veterinary Neurology. Oliner, J.E. and Lorenz, M.D. (Eds.), Saunders, Philadelphia, PA

14

Clinical Diagnostic Techniques in Ophthalmology

Eye is a very sensitive, delicate and unique organ. Its function may be affected with wide range of etiologies ranging from trauma, local and systemic infections, metabolic diseases to vision defects warranting an early and accurate diagnosis employing complete history, detailed ocular examination and or specialized diagnostic techniques such as Schirmer Tear Test (STT), Fluorescence Test, Ophthalmoscopy, Tonometry, Pachymetry, Retinoscopy and Gonioscopy etc.

Instruments for Ophthalmic Examination

- Finn off Transilluminator
- Pen torch
- Direct Ophthalmoscope
- Indirect fundoscopic lens (2.2 diopter lens)
- Schirmer tear test strips
- Fluorescein strips
- Tonometer
- Tropicamide (1%). Pupil dilatation should be done after Schirmer tear test and intraocular pressure (IOP) examination. It should not be used in dogs affected with glaucoma.
- Topical anesthetics (proparacaine 0.5%)
- Sterile eye wash.

Sequence of Complete Eye Examination

The ophthalmic examination should preferably be done in the following order for better results.

- Neuro-ophthalmic examination should be the first examination to be conducted to evaluate the different responses/ reflexes (menace response, dazzle reflex, papillary light response, palpebral reflex and vestibule-ocular reflex) and ocular movement.
- Second examination in sequence is the examination of anterior segment of the eye. It should be conducted with proper and adequate light source and magnification in a dark room.
- After examining anterior segment, Schirmer tear test (STT) should be conducted to evaluate tear production. This test is conducted before any topical medicine is instilled in the eye.
- Next diagnostic test in order after STT is tonometry to measure intraocular pressure. To be doubly sure in dogs with normal or low IOP values, the test may be repeated after dilatation of the pupil with tropicamide. Tropicamide induces mydriasis in 15-20 minutes lasting for 4-6 hours.
- Swabs for cytology and cultural examination, if indicated, are taken. This procedure is to be conducted prior to fluorescein stain.
- Next in order is fluorescein stain examination for detecting ulcers.
- It is followed by examination for tear break up time
- Fundus examination is conducted after dilating pupil using indirect ophthalmoscopy with a lens for an overview of the fundus. Direct ophthalmoscopy is better for evaluating lesions.

Ophthalmic Examination

For routine general inspection of the eyes, no sedation / anesthesia is required. It is better to perform general inspection in a dark room with low ambient light. Eyes should be examined for reflexes and responses, globe movement and position, vision, pupil size, palpebral lesion, moistness/ dryness of ocular surface, discharge and reflections.

Menace Response

Menace response (Figure128) in normal eye involves a blink and head aversion with threatening hand motion toward the eye without touching the patient or making a wind current. A normal menace response is indicative of vision and an intact facial nerve. A negative response is usually suggestive of blindness. Dogs with cerebellar lesions and normal vision also have negative menace response.This response involves the retina, optic nerve, chiasm and optic tract (afferent) as well as facial nerve (efferent). Care must be taken not to touch the whiskers or vibrissae, nor create an air current that could stimulate the cornea. Some normal cats will have a very weak or even absent menace response; in others the response will be brisk. Each side should be tested independently by covering one eye with the examiner's hand. A positive menace response allows the examiner to determine that at least some vision is present, but cannot assess quality or completeness of vision. Kittens do not develop a menace response until approximately 12 weeks of age.

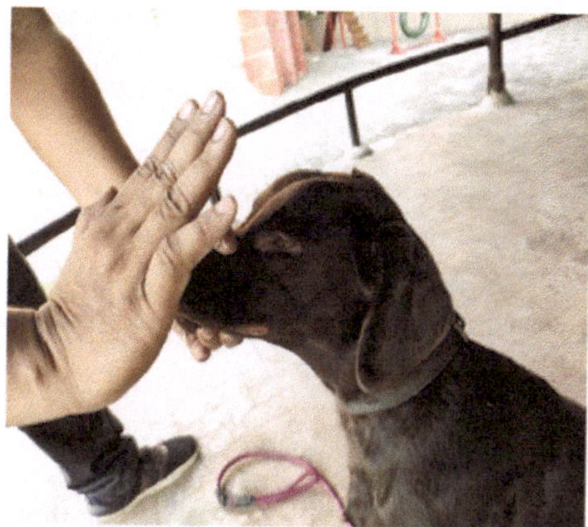

Figure 128: Performing a menace response test. The test is performed by waving a hand towards patient's face in a threatening manner. Normally it is associated with eye blinking.

Dazzle Reflex

A dazzle reflex involves blinking or partial blinking and head aversion in response to a bright light (Fin off Trans illuminator) being quickly shone on the eye. Negative response is poor prognostic indicator of vision. This reflex is subcortical and is thus not a test of vision. A dazzle reflex can be elicited at a much younger age than a menace response, essentially as soon as the eyelids open. Dazzle reflex is indicated to check for potential vision in cases having some opacity of ocular media as is seen in cases of cataract and hyphaema.

Palpebral Reflex

Palpebral reflex test (Figure129) is indicated in patients showing negative menace response test or dazzle reflex test. The test is performed by gently tapping/touching the eyelids at the medial and lateral canthi and observing a blink. In normal eyes, stimulation of medial and lateral canthus with gentle touch elicits a complete blink or closure of eye lids. A normal palpebral reflex test is indicative of an intact sensory (medial and lateral canthus branches of the trigeminal nerve) and motor pathway (facial nerve). A lack of blink in response to palpebral reflex suggests poor sensation or facial nerve paralysis.

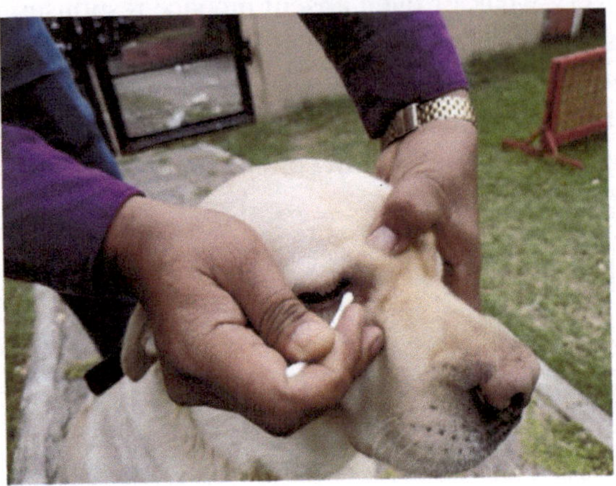

Figure 129: Testing of palpebral reflex in dog. The test is conducted by touching medial or lateral canthi and observing the blink response.

Pupil size and shape

The symmetry of size and shape of the pupil is evaluated by holding a torch at arm's distance and directing it toward the forehead so that both pupils are equally illuminated. The test in done in a room with normal room light followed by dimming of the room lights to recognize subtle anisocoria (difference in pupil size).

Pupillary Light Reflex (PLR)

A bright light is shone (Figure 130) into lateral aspect of each eye turn by turn. Constriction of the pupil of the eye(direct reflex) being stimulated by light and slightly less constriction or weak constriction of the pupil of the other unstimulated eye (indirect reflex) is the normal response. After few seconds wait for the pupils to return to resting size, the test is repeated on the other eye. The PLR is not a test of vision as blind animals (those with cataract or occipital cortex lesion) may have normal PLR and animals with normal vision (those with iris atrophy) may have negative PLR. Kittens at the time the eyelids open may have positive PLR. Some older cats may have mydriatic pupils with a weak or absent PLR due to iris sphincter muscle atrophy. Failure of pupil to constrict in response to bright light can be due to too weak light source; very much stressed animal with excessive sympathetic nerve stimulation; atrophy of iris muscle; extensive degeneration of retinal, optic nerve or optic tract; or dysfunction of oculomotor nerve (cranial nerve III).

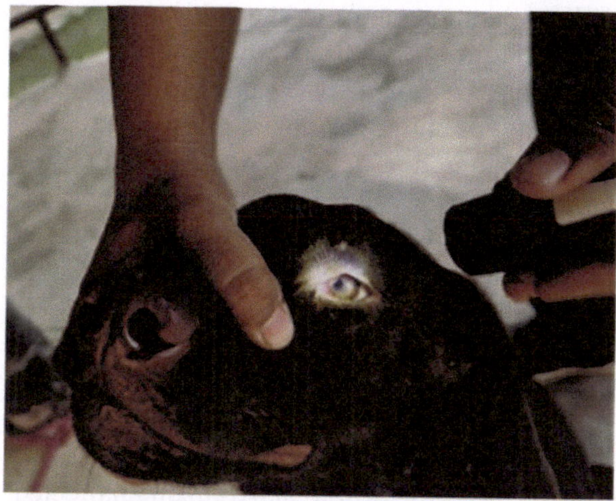

Figure 130: Performing a pupil light response test in a dog. The test is performed by shining a bright light into one eye and noting the constriction of pupil of the eye being tested as well as other eye also.

Examination of the anterior segment

Third eyelid, nasolacrimal puncta, conjunctiva, sclera, corneo-scleral limbus, tear film, cornea, anterior chamber, iris, pupil and lens are the constituents of the anterior segment. These parts should be examined using proper illumination (diffuse illumination, retro-illumination and trans-illumination with a slit beam). For diffuse illumination, Finnoff transilluminator can be used. The eye is examined from different angles under the light directed from a variety of contrasting angles. Retro-illumination is used to examine the transparent structures of the eye such as the tear film, cornea, anterior chamber, lens and vitreous. Trans-illumination is done using magnification and a slit beam.

Tonometry

Tonometry is a non-invasive technique used in clinical settings to measure intraocular pressure (IOP) indirectly. There are three types of tonometry viz. indentation, applanation and rebound tonometry. All these tonometry measure the bulbar tonus. Principles of indentation and applanation tonometry are based on Imbert-Flick law, which states that the external force (W) applied to spherical structure equals the pressure inside the spherical structure (Pt) multiplied by the area (A) that is flattened by the force. Rebound tonometry, on the other hand, relies on estimating the IOP by evaluating the kinematics of a probe that is electromagnetically shot against the cornea (Von Spiessen *et al.*, 2015). Applantation tonometry requires much co-operation from the patients.

Schiotz tonometer is used in indentation tonometry. When Schiotz tonometer (Figure 131) or Tono-Pen tonometer (Figure 131) is used to measure IOP, topical anesthesia is required. No anesthesia is required when rebound tonometer, Tono-Vet (Figure 131) is used for measuring IOP. Applantation tonometry is based on the principle that the force required to flatten a given area of cornea (sphere) is equal to the pressure within that sphere. Gentle handling of the patient is very much desirable to avoid inducing temporary increase in IOP. Normal values of intraocular pressure varies from 15 to 25 mm Hg in dogs and from 9 to 31 mm Hg in cats. Normally, IOP in both eyes of the same dog/ cat should not vary >20% (Miller and Bentley, 2015). Increase in IOP values beyond normal values (> 25 mm Hg) is suggestive of glaucoma, or orbital space occupying lesions such as neoplasia, cellulitis. Decrease in IOP (< 10 mm Hg) may be seen in old dogs and cats; and in cases of anterior uveitis. In keratitis, conjunctivitis and scleritis, the value of IOP may remain unaffected. Tonometry should be done in all cases with red eyes or in cases where there is a plan to administer atropine or tropicamide as these are contraindicated in cases of glaucoma.

Schiotz tonometer applies a rod of certain weight to the surface of the cornea (Figure 132). The distance that the rod indents the cornea is inversely related to the pressure within the eye. The distance the rod moves is reflected in the movement of a small metal tone arm across the number scale on the top of the instrument. This number is converted to mm Hg through the use of conversion scales for dogs and cats. When Schiotz tonometer or Tono-Pen tonometer is used to measure IOP, 1-2 drops of topical anesthesia (proparacaine) is instilled two times at 30 second interval .The tonometer is calibrated, before its application on the eye , in such a way that it is reading zero when applied on the metal button provided with the tonometer. The dog is restrained and positioned holding its muzzle high in such a way that the iris is parallel to the floor. This can be achieved in dorsal recumbency or in a sitting position with nose pointed upwards (Cho, 2020). A 5.5 g weight is applied on the piston of the tonometer and three readings are taken and averaged. The value is converted to mm Hg through the use of conversion table. Indentation technique using Schiotz tonometer should not be used in dogs with severely ulcerated cornea or granulation tissue formation (Heinrich, 2014).

Tono- Vet or Tono-Pen vet tonomters are based on applanation technique. Its basic principle is same as of indentation technique. Tonopen is a hand held applanation tonometer. In applanation tonometry, the force required to flatten a small ares of the cornea with tonometer tip is converted to IPO as mm Hg. This tonometer can be used in animals in any position. The tonometer should be perpendicular to the eye, so that tip is parallel to the corneal surface during the procedure. The tonometer is calibrated before use. Topical anesthesia (as described in Schiotz procedure) is instilled in to the eye. After 30 seconds eye lid is gently opened while the animal is held in sitting position with head right in midline. The Tono-Pen sensor must contact the axial cornea directly (ie, not at an angle), thus applanating the cornea at the sensor tip. This is done using a rapid and gentle touch that is repeated. Excessive pressure on the neck and excessive globe compression should be avoided. Reading are taken until the Tono-Pen's audible tone changes indicating that the average of three readings has been done.

Rebound tonometry is handy, portable and convenient technique with a lowest risk of corneal damage that measures IOP by using an induction coil to magnetize a small plastic tipped metal probe that is launched against the cornea. An induction current is created as the probe is rebound back to the instrument. Higher the IOP, faster the probe returns to its sleeve (Von Spiessen et al., 2015). No topical anesthesia is needed for the procedure (Heinrich, 2014). The instrument is held with the probe directed horizontally thus requiring appropriate positioning of patient's head. The tonometer is held at a 4-8mm distance from the eye surface to measure IOP. IOP is calculated from the value of induction current. A series of readings is taken, from which an average IOP is determined. The major disadvantage of this technique is that it difficult to use in recumbent patients.

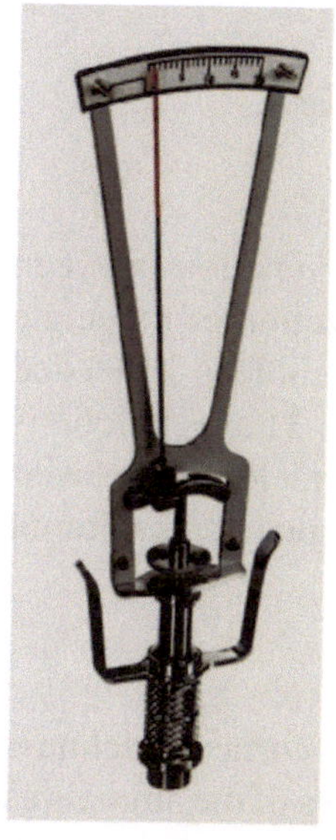

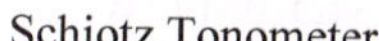

Schiotz Tonometer

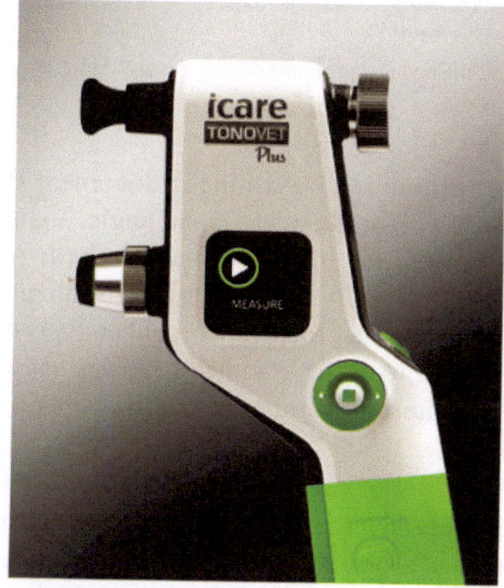

Tono-Vet Tonometer

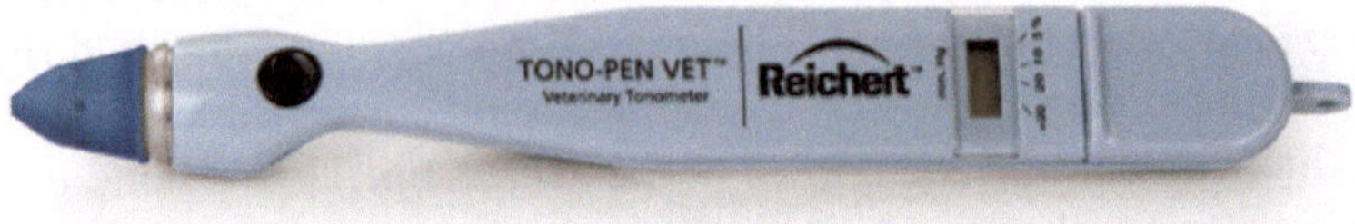

Tono-Pen Tonometer

Figure 131: Showing different types of tonometer. **A.** Schiotz tonometer. **B,** Tono-Vet tonometer. **C.** Tono-pen tonometer.

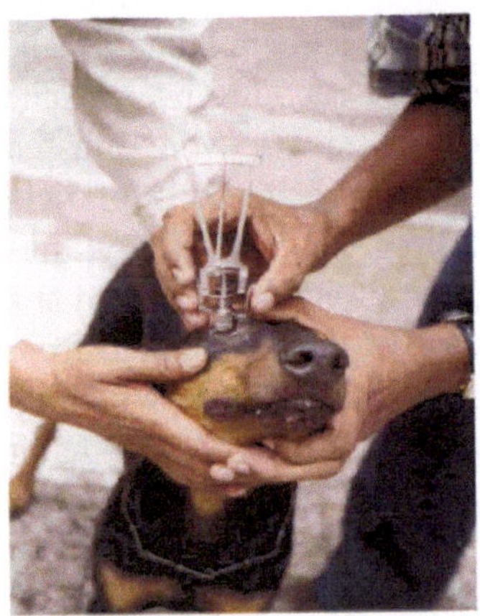

Figure 132: Measuring intraocular pressure of a dog using Schiotz tonometer.

Gonioscopy

Gonioscopy is the technique to examine iridocorneal (the junction between the iris and cornea/sclera) angle or drainage angle. Visualization of the angle in normal eyes is not feasible owing to scleral shelf. A goniolens is needed to refract the light and magnify the image for visualization. The technique is helpful in determining whether the iridocorneal angle is open, close, narrow or obstructed. It is possible to observe some of the drainage angle in cats without using a goniolens as anterior chamber in cats is deeper.

Pachymetry

Pachymetry is a simple, painless technique to measure the corneal thickness used in glaucoma. The corneal thickness varies among species of the animals as well as across corneal regions. In animals corneal thickness is usually between

0.5 and 0.8 mm. The measurement of corneal thickness is indicated in corneal transplantation, keratoconus screening, glaucoma, bulbous keratopathy and corneal edema.

Schirmer Tear Test (STT)

The Schirmer tear test was devised by Otto Schirmer, a German ophthalmologist, to measure ocular tear production and is generally indicated for the diagnosis of keratoconjunctivitis sicca (KCS).

The test is based on the principle of capillary action allowing water in the tears to travel along the length of the paper test strip in an identical fashion as a horizontal capillary tube. The rate of travel of the fluid along the test strip is proportional to the rate of tear production (Holly *et al.,* 1982).

Tear test strips are available in the market. The strips are with or without notch and are calibrated with a millimeter scale (Figure133). The strips of some manufacturers have a notch for easy placement besides calibration, and are also impregnated with a blue dye marking (Figure133) for an easy visualization of the result. No sedation or anesthesia is needed. The test should be conducted prior to instilling any topical drops (local anesthetic or fluorescein dye). Notched area of the strip is bent over 90°.The strip should not be touched at any other place except at notched end to avoid absorption of oils present on the skin of fingers of the examiner and consequently interfering with the passage of tears down the strip. The lower eyelid is slightly and gently pulled out. The notched section of the strip is inserted over the lower lateral eyelid margin into the conjunctival fornix for 60 seconds (Figure134). After 60 seconds the strip is taken out and the distance travelled by the tears on the test strip in sixty seconds is recorded.

In healthy dogs the normal values of the Schirmer tear test have been reported ranging from 20.4± 2.89 to 23.56± 3.98 mm/min (Hartly *et al.*, 2006; Visser *et al.*, 2017).The values of Schimer tear test in healthy cats are lower than that of dogs and are in the range of 13.7 ± 4.6 to 15.7 ± 3.7 mm/minute (Sebbag *et al.,* 2020). STT values of < 10 mm/minute in dogs are considered indicative of insufficient tear production warranting treatment. While STT values between 10 to 15 mm /min are considered lower values may or may not require treatment but constant monitoring is advised. Usually STT values between 15 to 25 mm /min are considered as normal in dogs. Keratoconjunctivitis sicca is not as common in cats as in dogs. In fact excessive tearing is more common in cats. STT values < 9 mm/min is considered consistent with KCS.

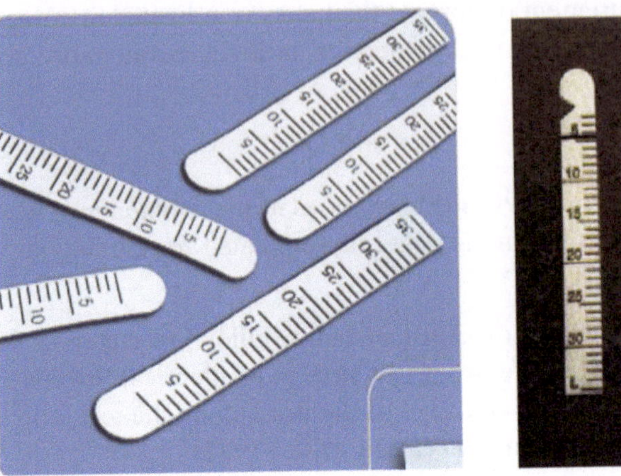

Figure 133: Schirmer tear test calibrated strips with or with out notch

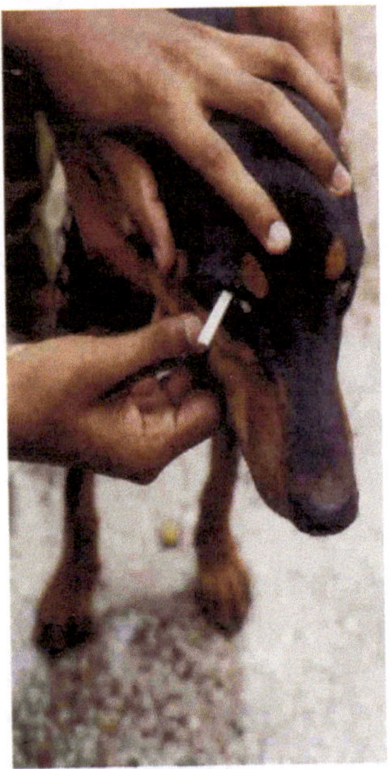

Figure 134: Placement of Schirmer tear test strip over the lower lateral eyelid margin into the conjunctival fornix.

Strip Meniscomerty

The strip meniscometry is a novel technique for quantitative measurement of tear volume in tear meniscus in 5 seconds. It is used to diagnose dry eyes. Strip meniscometry (SM) test was first used by Dogru *et al.* in 2006 for quantifying the tear volume in the tear meniscus (TM) in humans. Its applicability has also been reported in dogs and cats. The test has a strong correlation with the Schirmer test, tear film break-up time (BUT), and ocular surface vital staining scores. The SM tube testing strip possesses a tubular structure to induce the capillary action, which aids in tear absorption. It has three layers. The top and bottom layers comprise polyurethane tape and polyester tape respectively. The middle layer comprises polyurethane backing that forms a ditch along the longitudinal dimension. The tear absorption path is filled with an absorber made of nonwoven fabric (polyethylene terephthalate) facilitating a smooth and uniform absorption of the tears. The tip of the SMTube testing strip (SMTM strip- Fukushima-ken, Japan or I-Tear Test strip), is placed precisely at the edge of the lower tear meniscus without touching the eyelid or the cornea for 5 seconds and the result is immediately determined (Dogru *et al.*, 2006). Length of the blue stained tear column in the central membrane ditch (in millimeters) is considered as the meniscometry strip value for that eye in mm/5 s. SM TM values for normal dogs and cats have been reported as 9.66 ± 2.15 mm/5 s and10.50 ± 0.7 mm/5 s respectively (Rajaei *et al.*, 2017).

Fluorescein Eye stain Test

Fluorescein is a water soluble ophthalmic dye available as 1 to 2% sterile solution. Fluorescein impregnated paper strips (Figure 135) are also available. The strips can be moistened by a drop of sterile saline or local anesthetic. One drop is applied in the eye .The dye is highly hydrophilic and does not remain in contact with an intact corneal epithelium .Corneal ulceration causes breach in corneal epithelium exposing the stroma. When fluorescein dye is applied in cases of corneal abrasion/ulceration, the exposed stroma absorbs and retains fluorescein dye. A clear area at the base of the corneal defect is clearly marked (Figure136). Examination with blue light or Wood's lamp light greatly enhances fluorescein stain uptake. This test is conducted to detect corneal injuries/ ulcers, small foreign bodies or particles in the eyes, and tear break up time. It can also be used for the diagnosis of descemetocoele as descemetocoeles do not take up stain. Appearance of the dye in the mouth or at nares confirms nasolacrimal duct patency.

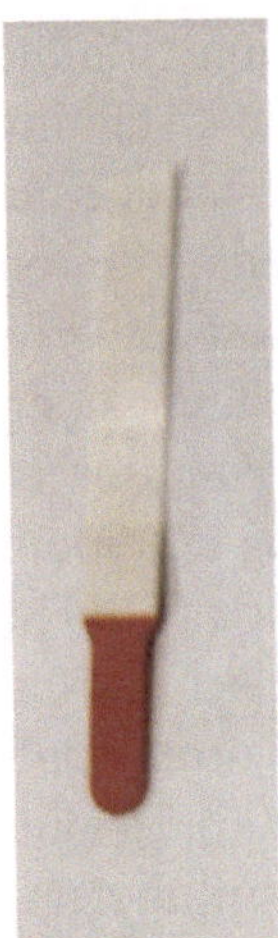

Figure 135: Fluorescein impregnated strip

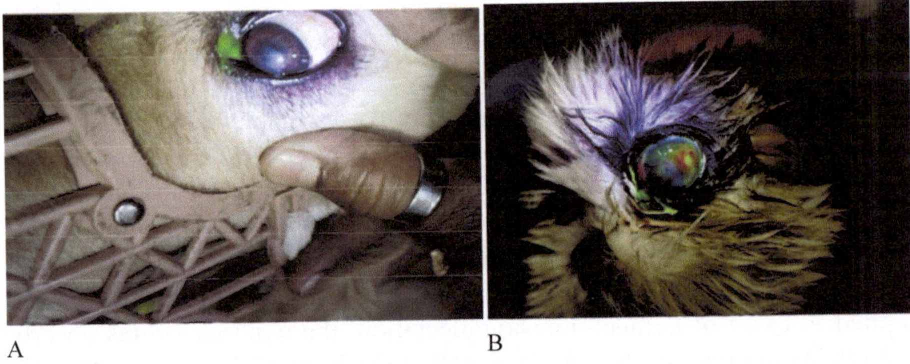

A B

Figure 136: Fluorescein eye stain test in dogs. The instilled stain in eyes is not retained by intact corneal epithelium **(A)**, while, the exposed stroma of cornea in corneal ulcers/abrasions absorbs and retains the stain giving the yellowish-green color to the lesion **(B)**.

Tear Break up Time (TBUT)

It is a non-invasive assessment of precorneal tear film stability and is frequently performed in cases of conjunctival hyperemia, chemosis, ocular discharge or keratitis. The fluorescein stain or fluorescein impregnated strip is lightly applied/touched to the dorsal bulbar conjunctiva .The animal is allowed to blink eye. The lights in the room are turned off. The eyelid is manually closed and then held open leaving the eye lid margin in contact with the globe. The cornea is examined under the cobalt blue light for dark spots (areas of drying) and time is counted in seconds from the time of opening of the eye lid until dark spots or lines appear in the fluorescein stain (Gelatt *et al.*,2011). The results of the test are highly variable. TBUT value in healthy dogs have been reported varying from 15 to 40 seconds (Saito and Kotani, 2001).

Seidel test

Fluorescein stain is applied to the eye as usual. Actively leaking lesions show a trail of aqueous through the fluorescein.

Examination of the Posterior Segment

Ophthalmoscopy

Ophthalmoscopy is the technique to examine the posterior segment of the eye. Ophthalmoscopes are of three types viz. direct ophthalmoscope, monocular indirect ophthalmoscope or indirect lens. Irrespective of ophthalmoscope being used, pupil dilatation is mandatory for the fundus examination. Pupil dilatation occurs around 15 minutes after instilling 1% tropicamide (1-2 drop). Degree and speed of dilatation can be enhanced by instilling a second drop after 5 minutes of the first dose.

(a) *Indirect Ophthalmoscopy:* A hand held lens is held at arm's length from the observer's eye and put next to the patient's eye (usually 20 to 30 dioptric). An inverted and reversed image is obtained that facilitates comparison of various regions of the fundus within a field. It is preferred as an initial scanning technique.

(b) *Direct Ophthalmoscopy:* The direct ophthalmoscope has a rheostat to adjust the brightness, colored filters, a slit beam for viewing elevations and depressions within the fundus, an illuminated grid that can be projected onto the fundus to measure lesions, and a set of lenses on a rotating wheel to change the depth of focus inside the eye. It provides an upright and magnified (15 to 17 times) image.

(c) *Monocular Indirect Ophthalmoscopy:* Monocular indirect ophthalmoscopes can be used with the same battery-powered handset as direct ophthalmoscopes. These ophthalmoscopes provide an image that is erect and have a moderate field of vision and magnification. They are comfortable with one hand

Optical coherence tomography (OCT)

It is a non- contact, non- invasive ophthalmic imaging technique that produces high-resolution images. OCT is often compared to B-scan ultrasonography but it relies upon reflections of light instead of dynamic echoes of ultrasound to yield a two-dimensional image of the retina. Optical coherence tomography system consists of fundus viewing unit, interferometer unit, computer display, control panel and color inkjet printer. In this technique there is no direct contact with tissue. The technique is safer to the patients as compared to fundus fluorescein angiography. The technique is of great help in identifying structures such as: epiretinal membranes, vitreoretinal tractions, accumulation of fluid in the sub retinal space or neurosensory detachments, retinal detachments.

Retinoscopy

The retinoscopy is indicated to evaluate the refractive status of the eyes. The instrument is held with one hand at a fixed distance from the eye. Light from retinoscope is shone into an eye and light reflected from the retina (retinoscopic reflex) is examined. Depending on the refractive error the retinal reflex moves in a certain way inside the pupil. Trial lenses can be used to measure the amount of movement that a retinal reflex has, so that the refractive error can be estimated accurately (Bracun *et al.*, 2014).

Ocular Ultrasonography

This is a non- invasive imaging technique having a great potential for visualizing retrobulbar and intraocular lesions, especially when globe examination is hindered due to swollen eye lids or opacities preventing direct clinical evaluation of structures caudal to opacities (Fielding, 2001) .A drop of topical anesthetic (proparacaine 0.5%)) is instilled in to eye. Ultrasound probe with sterile, water-soluble coupling gel is applied directly to the cornea or eyelids as the case may be. Ocular ultrasonography is indicated for the diagnosis of retinal separation, lens dislocation or rupture, vitreous degeneration or hemorrhage, asteroid hyalosis, synchysis scintillans, intraocular tumors or foreign bodies and getting fine-needle aspirates of orbital and ocular lesions .

Other Advance Tests

Computed tomography (CT scan) and magnetic resonance imaging (MRI) are valuable diagnostic aids for assessing structures of the eye (globe, orbit and surrounding structures) that cannot be visualized clinically. Magnetic resonance imaging is superior for assessing the globe and optic nerve and CT scan is better for evaluation of orbital bone and mineralized tissues. .

References

Bracun, A., Ellis, A.D. and Hall, C. (2014).A retinoscopic survey of 333 horses and ponies in the U.K. Vet. Ophthalmol. 17:90-96.

Cho, J. (2020). Ophthalmic examination. In Clinical Veterinary Advisor, Dogs and Cats. Cohn, L.A. and Cote, E. (Eds.). 4th edn. Elsevier. pp. 1137-1139.

Dogru, M., Ishida, K., Matsumoto, Y., Goto, E., Ishioka, M., Kojima, T., Goto, T., Saeki, M. and Tsubota,K.(2006). Strip meniscometry: a new and simple method of tear meniscus evaluation. *Invest. Ophthalmol. Vis. Sci.* 47: 1895–1901.

Fielding, J.A.(2001). The eye and orbit. In: Clinical Ultrasound.Meire, H.B. (ed.). 2nd edn. Churchill Livingstone, Edinburgh. pp. 938-964.

Gelatt, K.N., Ben-Shlomo, G., Gilger, B.C., Hendrix, D.V.H., Kern, T.J. and Plummer, C.E. (2021). The eye examination and diagnostic procedures. In: Veterinary Ophthalmology. Featherstone, H.J. and Heinrich, C.L. (eds). 6th edn. John Wiley and Sons Inc. pp 601–618.

Hartly, C., Williams, D. and Adams, V.J. (2006). Effect of age, gender, weight, and time of day on tear production in normal dogs. Vet. Ophthalmol. 9: 53–57.

Heinrich, C. (2014). The ocular examination. In BSAVA Manual of Canine and Feline Ophthalmology: Gould, D. and McLellan G. (Eds.) 3rd edn. British Small Animal Veterinary Association. pp. 1-23..

Holly, F.J., Lamberts, D.W. and Esquivel, E.D.(1982). Kinetics of capillary tear flow in the Schirmer strip. Curr. Eye Res. 2:57-70.

Miller, P.E and Bentley, E.(2015). Clinical signs and diagnosis of the canine primary glaucomas. Vet. Clinics: Small Anim. Pract. 45:1183-1212.

Rajaei, S.M., Mood, M.A., Asadi, A., Rajabian, M.R. and Aghajanpour, L.(2017). Strip meniscometry in dogs,cats and rabbits. Vet.Ophthalmol. 21: 210-213.

Saito, A. and Kotani, T. (2001). Estimation of lachrymal level and testing methods on normal Beagles. Vet. Ophthalmol. 4:7–11.

Sebbag, L., Uhl, L.K., Schneider, B., Hayes, B., Olds, J. and Mochel, J.P.(2020). Investigation of Schirmer tear test-1 for measurement of tear production in cats in various environmental settings and with different test durations. J. Am. Vet. Med. Assoc. 256(6), 681–686.

Visser, H.E., Toffemire, K.L., Love-Myers, K.R., Allbaugh, R.A., Ellinwood, N.M., Dees, D.D., Ben-Shlomo, G. and Whitley, R.D. (2017). Schirmer tear test I in dogs: Results comparing placement in the ventral vs. dorsal conjunctival fornix. Vet. Ophthalmol. 20:, 522–525.

Von Spiessen, L., Karck, J., Rohn, K., Meyer-Lindenberg, A. (2015). Clinical comparison of the TonoVet® rebound tonometer and the Tono-Pen Vet® applanation tonometerin dogs and cats with ocular disease: glaucoma or corneal pathology. Vet. Ophthalmol. 18, 20-27.